Complex Regional

Pain Syndrome

What Is The Evidence?

Internet Address: www.aadep.org

Veritas Medicus and the American Academy of Disability Evaluating Physicians and its authors and editors have consulted sources believed to be knowledgeable in their fields. Neither Veritas Medicus nor AADEP assume responsibility for use of the information contained in this publication. Neither Veritas Medicus nor AADEP shall be responsible for, and expressly disclaim liability for, damages of any kind arising out of the use of, or reference to, or reliance on, the content of this publication. This publication is for informational purposes only. Neither Veritas Medicus nor AADEP provide medical, legal, financial or other professional advice and readers are encouraged to consult a professional advisor for such advice.

The content of this publication represents the views of the authors and should not be construed to be the views or policies of either Veritas Medicus nor AADEP, or of the institutions with which the authors are affiliated, unless this is clearly specified.

Additional copies of this book may be ordered by accessing the links from the AADEP website @ www.aadep.org

ISBN 978-0-9961244-0-9

This book is self-published through Ingram Spark via Martin Occupational Medicine PC located @ www.mom-pc.com

All profits from the sale of this book will be given to the American Academy of Disability Evaluating Physicians for continuance of its mission to advance the science, prevention, evaluation, and management of disability.

Introduction

This paper was created as a result of a directive from Veritas Medicus, the Foundation of the American Academy of Disability Evaluating Physicians. The mission of Veritas Medicus is to change the behavior of physicians and medical support professionals through education, research, and other activities, and to advance the medical science of disability evaluation and for all purposes allowable and consistent with the provisions of Section 501(c)(3) of the Internal Revenue Code.

One of the core activities of Veritas Medicus is to service the general public, public and private educational systems, medical boards and state and federal governmental agencies. Veritas Medicus provides evidence-based graduate and continuing medical education programs to qualify medical professionals and to change the behavior of both medical and non-medical professionals to meet the needs of the public in the practice of the medical science of disability prevention, evaluation, rehabilitation and treatment, as well as disability consultation and management; and by developing educational programs and training programs to support the medical practice of disability evaluation, and to interpret and develop the skill to use existing and future pertinent resources, such as Guides, guidelines, applicable governmental rules and regulations, established protocols, and medical evidence correctly.

We would like to acknowledge the prior work that prior AADEP authors gave towards the CRPS paper published in the Journal in 2002. Pain Med. 2002 Sep;3(3):274-88.

As medicine changes, we should be aware that many forces mold the behavior of physicians and other ancillary practitioners and are oftentimes not based in scientific discipline. While recognizing the disability epidemic in the United States cannot go unchecked, we offer this work as a comprehensive treatise on the construct of Complex Regional Pain Syndrome. Our hope is that it is recognized, implemented and used as a springboard for change into the future. Our patients, our colleagues, the house of medicine, and the nations of the world deserve it.

Of note, wherever in this text you see the term "CRPS", the reference is to the construct known as Complex Regional Pain Syndrome.

About the Authors

Douglas W Martin MD, FAADEP, FACOEM, FAAFP is an occupational medicine physician practicing in Sioux City, Iowa. Originally trained in Family Medicine, he has spent greater than 20 years in clinical based musculoskeletal injury care. While focused on treatment of these conditions, he is also involved in medico-legal evaluations and is keenly interested in the bio-psychosocial implications of claim behavior and patient outcomes. He is a Past President of the Iowa Academy of Family Physicians and the American Academy of Disability Evaluating Physicians. He has held many positions within the American College of Occupational and Environmental Medicine. While not in the clinic or volunteering to teach at CME courses, he spends time officiating football, supporting his athletic children in sports events, and serving the Boy Scouts of America (once an Eagle, always an Eagle). Dr. Martin served as the lead editor for this work.

Robert J. Barth, PhD is a fellow of the National Academy of Neuropsychology for making significant contributions to science and practice. He has created educational publications and programs regarding the construct of complex regional pain syndrome at the invitation of AADEP, the American Medical Association, the American Academy of Orthopedic Surgeons, the European Union of Medicine in Assurance and Social Security, the North American Spine Society, the Journal of Hand Surgery / American Society for Surgery of the Hand, the National Association of Workers' Compensation Judiciary, and other professional organizations and government entities internationally. He has participated in the review and creation of guidelines regarding this construct at the invitation of the American Academy of Neurology, the American Medical Association, the American College of Occupational and Environmental Medicine, and the Official Disability Guidelines. Health science organizations and government entities have also invited Dr. Barth to create a variety of other educational publications and programs which focus on the scientific knowledge base regarding chronic pain.

Trang Nguyen MD, PhD is board certified in Family Medicine and is a practicing board eligible Occupational Medicine physician in Cincinnati, Ohio. She completed the Doctoral Degree in Epidemiology at the University of Cincinnati, College of Medicine. Dr. Nguyen is a clinician and a researcher. She was an Assistant Professor at UT Southwestern Medical School at Dallas, Department of Family Medicine. Dr. Nguyen is an author and a member of the Spine Editorial Board. She is also a member of the ODG Editorial Advisory Board. Her interests include evidence based medicine, cost effectiveness research, lumbar spine treatment, pain interventions, and opioid treatments.

David C. Randolph M.D., PhD, M.P.H is an active Occupational Medicine physician in Cincinnati, Ohio. He has been in practice for 25 years. He is the Past President of the American Academy of Disability Evaluating Physicians. He was a contributor to the AMA 5th Edition Guides and a reviewer of the 6th edition. His Doctoral Degree is in Epidemiology from the University Of Cincinnati College Of Medicine. His main interest is the study and provision of safe and effective care for injured workers. He is a member of the Alpha Omega Alpha Honor Medical Society and is an Eagle Scout.

Russell L. Travis, M.D., FACS, FAADEP is a neurosurgeon currently serving as Associate Medical Director at Cardinal Hill Rehabilitation Hospital in Lexington, Kentucky. He is Past President of the American Academy of Disability Evaluating Physicians, American Association of Neurological Surgeons, and the Neurosurgical Society of America. He holds a volunteer faculty appointment within the University of Kentucky Physical Medicine and Rehabilitation Department. Dr. Travis serves on numerous advisory boards and has been a contributing author or reviewer for the Official Disability Guidelines, the American College of Occupational & Environmental Medicine Practice Guidelines Chapters on Spine and Pain, and the AMA Guides to the Evaluation of Permanent Impairment, 6th edition.

James B Talmage, M.D. is an orthopedic surgeon by training. He is Board Certified in Orthopedic Surgery and in Emergency Medicine. He currently practices Occupational Medicine in Cookeville, TN. He also serves as Assistant Medical Director for the State of Tennessee Division of Workers' Compensation. He is an Adjunct Associate Professor of Occupational Medicine at Meharry Medical College in Nashville. He is a Past President of the American Academy of Disability Evaluating Physicians (AADEP). Since 1992 he has lectured over 700 times to physician audiences in courses sponsored by AADEP, AAOS, ACOEM, SEAK, and multiple other organizations. He does unpaid peer review of articles submitted to 2 medical journals. He is a Co-Editor of the textbook published by the American Medical Association on Causation and the textbook on Work Ability. He has helped author many AMA products on impairment rating. He is a paid consultant to the Federal Motor Carrier Safety Administration (FMCSA) and National Institute of Occupational Safety and Health (NIOSH)

Disclosures

The authors of this work were selected by the Veritas Medicus Board of Directors and approved by the Board of Directors of the American Academy of Disability Evaluating Physicians as experts in their reflective fields and renowned reviewers of the medical literature on the topic of CRPS.

None of the authors received an honorarium for their work on this project. The budget for this work included funds to cover travel and incidental expenses for the authors to attend one in-person meeting and to cover expenses for teleconferences. The budget also included expenses for editorial review conducted by Tracey Pick, ARNP who practices occupational medicine and who holds a graduate degree in English who has provided editorial assistance on a number of medical writing projects in her career.

No author has a conflict of interest. Each author is primarily a clinician and has no vested interest in any product or service that would result in financial gain as a result of participation in this project.

TABLE OF CONTENTS

Executive Summary

Complex Regional Pain Syndrome (CRPS) is a construct that was created in the mid-1990s by a group of invited physicians in an attempt to describe a constellation of symptoms that were previously attributed to causalgia and reflex sympathetic dystrophy.

The impetus for such creation was historically based upon a desire to describe variable upper and lower extremity problems that were first identified during the US Civil War but have been the subject of considerable debate and nomenclature changes for over 100 years.

As a construct, CRPS was developed without a gold standard diagnostic benchmark. Over time, the criteria for the diagnosis of CRPS has been changed with little if any attention paid to the requisite history and physical examination application to the process of development of a differential diagnosis.

Basic science research focused upon investigating the true cause of CRPS has created a wide range of hypotheses. None of these hypotheses have been shown to be consistent amongst patient populations and a cause has not been specifically identified or accepted within the medical community.

Without a gold standard, research conducted upon patients who have been given this diagnosis is subject to criticism because of patient selection, inappropriate labelling, and a lack of focus on a differential-diagnostic-driven medical investigation into other common causes of limb symptoms. Treatments that have been advocated for patients with CRPS have focused upon pain relief but there has been little attention paid to functional recovery.

As CRPS predominates as a diagnosis in cases where patients are involved in medico-legal claims for compensation, questions arise regarding its validity as a true medical issue. Psychological and social issues seem to drive the making of this diagnosis by physicians who struggle with the patient who has ongoing limb symptomatology that does not respond to conventional treatment.

When in the course of treating patients who have been given this diagnosis, the physician should be cognizant of the inherent problems that the CRPS construct creates regarding disability issues. A focus should be turned towards resumption of normal activity of the painful limb in question, which includes a goal of return to normal work within the context of a workers compensation claim.

When the physician is confronted with a claimant who has been given this diagnosis and is asked to provide an impairment rating, despite the AMA Guides having specific sections devoted to the construct of CRPS, it is best to apply the process of impairment rating determination similar to that of other painful limb conditions without creating a "special place" for CRPS.

The development of the CRPS construct has overall proven to be a failure. As such, the term should be abandoned and effort should turn toward determining what this is as opposed to describing what it is not.

Section 1

Antecedents to and the Creation of the CRPS Construct

Several sources attribute the creation of the term "causalgia" (Greek *kausos* + *algos* = "burning" "pain") to Silas Weir Mitchell in 1864 as the first attempt to describe the pain syndrome that would eventually morph into the term CRPS.[1,2] However, Potts described burning pain and atrophy in an injured extremity as early as 1700.[3] Denmark, Hamilton and Paget also described certain features of burning limb pain in their writings.[4-6] Mitchell observed that Civil War soldiers sustaining major nerve injuries affecting their limbs sometimes experienced long-lasting pain that was burning in quality.[7]

It is interesting to note that the historical development of the term "causalgia" and its proper attribution may very well be as ambiguous and controversial as the modern term CRPS is today. While Mitchell wrote eloquently about the symptoms and signs that these civil war soldiers were experiencing in the book *Gunshot Wounds and Other Injuries of Nerves*[7], he never used the term "causalgia" until a second book was written in 1872 entitled *Injuries of The Nerves and Its Consequences*.[8] Even in this second book, the term "causalgia" is not defined and is included within the text as though the term had been commonplace. What then happened between 1864 and 1872?

In a little known article contained within the *United States Sanitary Commission Memoirs* from 1867, Mitchell states the following:

> "Causalgia - There is, however, one species of pain arising out of nerve wounds which had never been described except by my colleagues and myself, although the state of skin which is usually found with it had been spoken of by Mr. Paget, who seems to have seen it only in association with common neuralgic pains. In writing of this peculiar kind of suffering, I felt that it would be well to give it some more convenient name than merely 'burning pain', and, in accordance with the suggestion of my friend, Professor Robley Dunglison, I have therefore adopted the term Causalgia as being both descriptive and convenient."[9]

There can, therefore, be no doubt that Weir Mitchell was the first person to use the term "causalgia." Credit for the origin of the term must properly be accorded to Dunglison. In 1874, Dunglison's son edited his original Medical Dictionary, to include the term "causalgia."[10]

The next major milestone in the development of the construct occurred in 1900 when Paul Sudek made the discovery that osteoporosis can occur in acute focal limb disorders.[11] Hence, the term "Sudek's atrophy," which in some texts was used as a synonym for causalgia.

The French vascular surgeon Leriche postulated that the sympathetic nervous system mediated pain responses. Leriche first described the surgical procedure of sympathectomy in 1916 as an option for controlling limb pain.[12] Shortly thereafter, in 1926, his writings contained the observation that sympathetic nerve root dysfunction could be the cause of limb pain. In a remarkable, yet somewhat off-handed comment, he provided fast forward insight into the modern day adjustments to diagnostic criteria by suggesting that trauma may not be the only precursor to such dysfunction.[13]

DeTakats was the first to use the term "reflex dystrophy" in 1937. His hypothesis was that there was some form of reflex mechanism involving the nervous system.[14] It is interesting to note that 6 years later, he, along with Miller, would suggest an explicitly psychogenic component to the construct, again illustrating the divergence of causation philosophies which remains pervasive today.[15] Finally, in 1946 Evans was the first to use the term "reflex sympathetic dystrophy".[16] Reflex sympathetic dystrophy, or RSD, is a phrase that is still used today. The term was used because DeTakats postulated that trauma that generated activity in afferents sets up a reflex in the spinal cord which stimulated activity in the sympathetic efferents. This in turn resulted in dystrophic changes in the periphery of the limb. Remarkable for the time, the speculation that central changes in the spinal cord could spread and also affect the brain held true amongst medical scientists for a few decades.

As time went on, a variety of reports indicated that there may be a milder form of the syndrome.[17] Additionally, speculation grew that its development might be possible without trauma to a nerve.[18] As a result, two terms became used more by default than by science; "causalgia" meaning that the syndrome was due to a nerve trauma, and "reflex sympathetic dystrophy" indicating similar symptoms when no nerve trauma was found.

As is indicated in Schott's review of the disorder in 2007, debates and lack of scientific validation regarding major versus minor forms and the presence, or lack thereof, of involvement of the sympathetic nervous system set the scene for "nosological chaos".[1] Indeed, as time progressed, approximately 80 different names for this disorder have now appeared in English language literature. As late as 1986, the International Association for the Study of Pain (IASP) had paradoxically simultaneously published two different definitions for the condition called "causalgia" and continued to perpetuate that sympathetic involvement was necessary for the disorder "reflex sympathetic dystrophy".[1]

Having come to the realization that exponential descriptive divergences are not helpful in the science of medicine, the IASP created an invitation only panel in an attempt to re-direct the entropy.[19] The committee created the newly derived phrases CRPS Type I and CRPS Type II which were created to replace the prior terms reflex sympathetic dystrophy and causalgia respectively. Several authors have been critical of this process as well as the terminology. Barth has indicated that the creation of CRPS has created a level of intentional ambiguity.[20] Schott has questioned why the words were chosen, citing that there is nothing more "complex" about this pain compared to other difficult to characterize pain syndromes. Schott also argues that there is nothing "regional" about it, given the fact that the pain spreads. He notes that the very use of the term "pain" is perplexing as it may range from trivial to overwhelming.[1] Borchers has described the current term as "arbitrary".[21] As a result, there has been an ever-increasing call to revisit the syndrome in its entirety, with at least one author in a major medical journal calling for a comprehensive re-analysis in 2014.[22]

Section 1 References

1. Schott GD. Complex? Regional? Pain? Syndrome? Practical Neurology 2007; 7: 145–157

2. Weinberger M, Brannnagan III T., Complex Regional Pain Syndrome in Merritt's Neurology, 12th Edition. Philadelphia, JB Lippincott. 520

3. Richards RL (1967). "The Term 'Causalgia'". Medical History 11 (1): 86–90.

4. Denmark, A., Med. Chir. Trans., Lond., 1819, 4, 48.

5. Hamilton, J., Dubl. J. med. Sci., 1838, 13, 38.

6. Paget, J., Med. Times Gaz., 1864, 1, 331.

7. Mitchell, S. W., Morehouse, G. R. and Keen, W. W., Gunshot Wounds and other Injuries of Nerves, Philadelphia, J. B. Lippincott, 1864.

8. Mitchell, S. W. Injuries of Nerves and Their Consequences. Philadelphia, J. B. Lippincott, 1872

9. Mitchell, S. W. 'On the Diseases of Nerves, Resulting from Injuries', in Contributions relating to the causation and prevention of disease, and to camp diseases, ed. Austin Flint, United States Sanitary Commission Memoirs, New York, 1867.

10. Dunlingson, R. A Dictionary of Medical Science, London, J. & A. Churchill, 1874

11. Sudeck P. U¨ber die akute entzu¨ndliche Knochenatrophie. Arch Klin Chir 1900;62:147–56.

12. Leriche R. De la causalgie envisage´e comme une ne´vrite du sympathique et de son traitement par la de´nudation et l'excision des plexus nerveux pe´ri arte´riels. Presse Me´d 1916;24:178–80

13. Leriche R., Leriche P., Thérapeutique chirurgicale. Vol. III (Abdomen et Organes génito-urinaires). Vols. I and II in the press. Royal 8vo. Pp. 646. 1926. Paris: Masson et Cie. Unbound, Fr. 50; bound, Fr. 60

14. de Takats, G. Reflex dystrophy of the extremities. Arehs. Surgery, 34: 939–956, 1937

15. de Takats, G. Post-traumatic dystrophy of the extremities. Arehs. Surgery, 46: 469–479, 1943.

16. Evans JA. Reflex sympathetic dystrophy. Surg Gynecol Obstet 1946;82:36–43.

17. Bonica, J.J. Causalgia and other reflex sympathetic dystrophies. In J.J. Bonica et al. (eds.), Advances in pain research and therapy. New York, 1979.

18. Hübner, L. Das Sudeck-Syndrom. Der Landarzt, 3: 651–657, 1957.

19. Stanton-Hicks M, Janig W, Hassenbusch S, Haddox JD, Boas R, Wilson P. Reflex sympathetic dystrophy: changing concepts and taxonomy. Pain. 1995;63:127–33

20. Barth RJ. A Historical Review of Complex Regional Pain Syndrome in the "Guides Library" and Broader Issues Raised by That History. The Guides Newsletter. November/December 2009. American Medical Association

21. Borchers AT, Gershwin ME. Autoimmun Rev. 2014 Mar;13(3):242–65.

22. Basler, MH. BMJ 2014;348:g4029 doi: 10.1136/bmj.g4029 (Published 24 June 2014)

Section Two

Evolutionary Thoughts and the Application of Science

CRPS is a syndrome. A syndrome is a collection of symptoms and signs that are seen together in recognizable patterns; and that have no current known explanation or pathophysiology. Once science determines pathophysiology, syndromes are typically renamed. This is how "Down's syndrome" became Trisomy 21.

Patients with CRPS-like presentations typically have pain, and usually the pain is in one limb. The pain is not explained by another condition. The pain is not consistent with injury to or disease of a single peripheral nerve, multiple peripheral nerves, the brachial or the lumbosacral plexus, a nerve root or multiple nerve roots, the spinal cord (neuropathic pain), or joint, tendon, ligament, or muscle conditions (nociceptive pain).

The pain in CRPS is usually described as "burning" (suggesting it is neuropathic). It is classically described as disproportionate to any inciting event that may be associated with its onset.

In addition to pain, patients with CRPS-like presentations frequently have:

- Sensory symptoms: hyperesthesia and allodynia. This might suggest peripheral nerve, thalamic, and/or cortical involvement.

- Vasomotor symptoms: asymmetric limb color and limb temperature, assumed to reflect altered blood flow. This might suggest hypothalamic and/or sympathetic nervous system involvement

- Sudomotor symptoms: asymmetric edema or sweating. This might suggest hypothalamic and/or sympathetic nervous system involvement.

- Motor symptoms: weakness, tremor, or dystonia. This might suggest cortical, basal ganglia, and/or cerebellar involvement.

- Trophic symptoms: changes in growth and/or appearance of skin, fingerprints, nails, etc.

CRPS is probably a combination of many different conditions with similar symptom presentations. CRPS is classically subdivided into 2 sub-types, Type I and Type II. Type I occurs following injury with known nerve involvement (e.g. fracture, contusion, etc.). Type II occurs following an objectively documentable nerve injury. Similar presentations may occur spontaneously, although much less commonly. Therefore, trauma is not absolutely necessary. Reported series vary in how close in time the CRPS symptoms and signs must appear in relation to a potentially inciting traumatic event for the two to be considered associated.

Multiple names have been used during the three centuries in which this condition has been discussed by physicians. Beerthuizen's systematic review in 2009 found 72 names.[1] A theory to explain CRPS-like presentations has arisen as medical science progressed and new understanding of anatomy, physiology, neurology, biochemistry, immune function, and injury healing develop, permitting a new method of research. Discussed in the subsequent section on pathophysiology, no theory has been proven to apply to all cases. This is probably because many different rare conditions with similar presentations are being "lumped" together as a single entity, currently called CRPS.

American physicians may be skeptical once they are aware that, in reported CRPS patients seeking treatment, 54-81% of U.S. cases have treatment funded by U.S. workers' compensation insurance, even though less than 10% of U.S. injuries occur on the job and have workers' compensation coverage.[2]

CRPS occurs in Europe[3] and Asia[4], which are areas that don't have the US system of health care or the US system of workers' compensation. In the only 2 published prospective epidemiologic studies, CRPS-like presentations were more common in the Netherlands than in Minnesota[3,5] In addition, CRPS occurs in children. Thus, the U.S. workers' compensation is not a necessary prerequisite for a CRPS-like presentation.

Some CRPS-like presentations have been documented to be due to malingering and factitious disorder, complicating the search for pathophysiology.[6] Most reported case series do not include a deliberate search for malingering and factitious disorders in the patients comprising the series.

The original descriptions were of what today we call CRPS Type II. This follows a significant peripheral nerve injury. The original theories of pathophysiology involved an abnormal neurologic reflex involving pain signal carrying afferent peripheral nerve and sympathetic efferent nerves, so the old name of "reflex sympathetic dystrophy" seemed to make sense to some. However, over time it became clear there was no documented reflex. While some patients responded to sympathetic blocks or surgical sympathectomy, most CRPS-like patients did not have evidence that the sympathetic nervous system was involved in their pain syndrome. Hence, the name "Reflex Sympathetic Dystrophy," has fallen out of favor.

Current theories center on peripheral nerve sensitization and central nervous system sensitization and/or reorganization, due to genetic, autoimmune, and other unknown influences.

Until there is an objective way to separate all CRPS-like patients from those with other chronic pain syndromes, or until there is a way to separate many of the patients with CRPS like illness into objectively diagnosable subgroups, scientific understanding of this illness will remain primitive. Research continues.

Section 2 References

1. Beerthuizen A, van't Spijker A, Huygen FJMP, et al. Is there an association between psychological factors and Complex Regional Pain Syndrome Type I (CRPS) in adults? A Systematic Review. Pain 2009; 145: 52-9

2. [Chapter 11, Conditions of Uncertain Pathophysiology – Acute and Chronic Pain. In Melhorn, JM, Ackerman WE, Talmage JB, Hyman MH. *AMA Guides to the Evaluation of Disease and Injury Causation, 2nd Edition.* American Medical Association, Chicago, 2013

3. De Mos M, deBruijn AGJ, Huygen FJPM et al. The incidence of complex regional pain syndrome: a population-based study. Pain. 2007, 129:12–20

4. Choi YS, Lee MG, Lee HM, et al. Epidemiology of Complex Regional Pain Syndrome: A Retrospective Chart Review of 150 Korean Patients. J Korean Med Sci 2008; 23: 772-5

5. Sandroni P, Benrud-Larson LM, McClelland RL, Low PA. Complex regional pain syndrome type 1: incidence and prevalence in Olmsted county, a population-based study. Pain 2003; 103: 199-207

6. Ochoa JL, Verdugo RJ. Neuropathic pain syndrome displayed by malingerers J Neuropsychiatry Clin Neurosci. 2010 Summer; 22(3): 278–286

Section 3

Critical Analysis of the
IASP and Budapest Criteria
Study Design and Statistics

There are a total of four *original* publications on IASP and Budapest Criteria. The diagnosis of CRPS is based on the research findings of these four articles. They are summarized below:

Article One: The first article "IASP Diagnostic Criteria for Complex Regional Pain Syndrome: A Preliminary Empirical Validation Study" was published in 1998.[1] This study reports the results and analyses of 18 consecutive RSD patients and 30 diabetic neuropathy patients. The authors noted the original diagnosis was RSD but these patients do meet the IASP clinical diagnostic criteria for CRPS. It is not clear if this is CRPS Type 1 or CRPS Type 2. The time frame that patients are recruited for the study is not discussed.

Table 1. IASP Diagnostic Criteria for CRPS
The diagnosis of CRPS consists of the presence of: 1. An initiating noxious events or a cause of immobilization.   2. Continuing pain, allodynia or hyperalgesia with which pain is disproportionate to any inciting event.   3. Evidence at some time of edema, changes in skin blood flow, abnormal sudomotor activity in the region of pain.   4. This diagnosis is precluded by the existence of conditions that would otherwise account for the degree of pain and

In the results section of the article, Tables 2, 3, 4 and 5 listed sensitivity, specificity, and positive and negative predictive values of the criteria to make the diagnosis of CRPS. However, raw data to support these calculations is not provided. Results cannot be reproduced based on the limited information provided.

The authors concluded

> *"the diagnostic criteria of CRPS are intentionally broad to capture all patients with pain associated with dysautonomic*

features. The diagnosis of CRPS does not require any laboratory test or report of symptom relief following nerve block. CRPS diagnostic criteria are based chiefly on the patient's self-report and quasi-objective measures (subjective opinion of the examining physician)".

Furthermore, the criteria that describe the dysautonomic feature, probably the cardinal feature of these disorders, is overly vague.

"Evidence at some time (Criteria 3), which may be interpreted to mean the presence of one, several, or all dysautonomic sign being evident on the initial, past, or future examinations; for the present study, the diagnosis of CRPS required the presence of at least one sign on the initial physical examination."

The authors acknowledged that there were inherent problems with utilization of these rules and called for revision to them.

"The results of the present study suggest that the existing decision rules may lead to over diagnosis of CRPS, and therefore, these rules should be modified."

The author reported one of the limitations of this study is that the

"small sample size from a single investigator may not be a representation of the overall patient population with CRPS and diabetic neuropathy. An inherent problem in all diagnostic validation research in CRPS is that there is no gold standard against which validity can be judged. Given that the CRPS group was defined in the present study using strict interpretation of the published criteria #3 and #4, the present study made an assumption that was appropriate to define CRPS by using the specified criteria. Thus a strict interpretation of the current CRPS criteria was treated as an operationally defined gold standard for the purpose of this study. Recommendations based on these results must be considered in the context of this assumption."

The above statements summarized the underlying problems with all diagnoses of CRPS. The diagnosis is made based on assumption, self-reported symptoms, and subjective opinion of the examining physician. There is no gold standard to validate the diagnosis. Conclusions of studies are based on small sample size with no randomization. Analyses are provided with incomplete data.

Article 2- The second article "Complex regional pain syndrome: are the IASP diagnostic criteria valid and sufficiently comprehensive?"[2] was published in 1999. This study included a series of 123 patients reportedly meeting IASP criteria for CRPS from 7 US centers. Subject selection, time frame of subject recruitment and the number of CRPS Type I vs. CRPS Type II patients are not provided.

This study discussed the correlation between signs, symptoms, pain duration, block responsiveness, test results and internal validity of diagnostic criteria. It should be noted Table 3 within the article only has 5 variables with statistically significant correlation. These variables have weak correlation. The remaining variables have no statistical significance with weak to poor correlation. In other words, the observed effects could be due to chance.

The authors noted the sample size for the various objective test results are limited and results should be treated as *preliminary* findings.

Article 3- The third article was also published in 1999, "External validation of IASP diagnostic criteria for Complex Regional Pain Syndrome and propose research diagnostic criteria".[3] This study was designed to evaluate the external validity of IASP CRPS criteria and to evaluate the proposed research modifications of the CRPS criteria. This study included 117 CRPS patients and 43 patients with non-CRPS neuropathic pain consisting of diabetic neuropathy, polyneuropathy, post herpetic neuralgia, and radiculopathy.

Electro diagnostic studies were available in the "subset of CRPS patients, which if used as diagnostic criterion, would have led to the diagnosis of CRPS Type I in approximately two thirds of the sample". "*The remaining analyses did not separate these diagnostic subcategories.*" Based on the above statements, it is unclear how many patients have CRPS Type I and CRPS Type II. It appears CRPS Type I and CRPS Type II are considered the same and are analyzed as a single group.

Table 2 in the article presents sensitivity and specificity of the different IASP and research criteria. No raw data was provided for the reported sensitivity and specificity. In summary, due to the lack of raw data provided, the sensitivity and specificity provided in table 2 cannot be reproduced.
More importantly, presently there is no gold standard test to confirm the diagnosis of CRPS. Without this confirmation, the true positive and the calculation of sensitivity is not possible.

Sensitivity is defined as

$$\frac{\text{True Positive}}{\text{True positive + False Negative}}$$

Figure 1 describes the positive predictive power and negative predictive power for the proposed research criteria decision rule. The article discussed positive predictive power based on the assumption of a 25% prevalence of CRPS. The prevalence and the accuracy of diagnosing true positive CRPS remains unclear in the literature. I would note for this particular study, 117 CRPS patients are reported from multiple centers. It is unclear how many centers are involved in recruiting 117 subjects over what period of time. This small sample size (n = 117) does not support the high prevalence assumed in the study. Subject selection bias is a concern. It is unclear why there are more CRPS subjects compared to the number of non-CRPS neuropathic pain patients (n = 43) when the prevalence of diabetic neuropathy, polyneuropathy, post herpetic neuralgia, and radiculopathy is much higher than CRPS.

Article 4- The final article is from 2010 entitled "Validation of propose diagnostic criteria (the "Budapest criteria") for Complex Regional Pain Syndrome.[4]

The authors noted "current IASP diagnostic criteria for CRPS have *low specificity, potentially leading to over diagnosis.*"

This study is a validation study comparing the current (at the time) IASP diagnostic criteria for CRPS to the new Budapest criteria regarding diagnostic accuracy. Sample sizes include 113 CRPS Type I and 47 non-CRPS neuropathic pain patients. IASP criteria is reported with diagnostic sensitivity of 1.00 with poor specificity of 0.41. Poor specificity can lead to increased false positive diagnoses.

The Budapest clinical criteria is reported to have sensitivity of 0.99 and specificity of 0.68. It appears that CRPS Type I patients are analyzed with the small proportion of CRPS Type II (13%) patients. This is inaccurate as CRPS Type I and CRPS Type II patients are different clinically. There is no gold standard test to confirm the true positive patient with CRPS. Therefore, it is not possible to calculate sensitivity.

The number of CRPS patients is reported as 113 and non-CRPS patients is 47. Subject selection was not described. It is unclear why there are less non-CRPS patients compared to the CRPS patients when the prevalence of non-CRPS diagnoses are much more common.

Table 3 provided sensitivity, specificity, positive and negative predictive values with the assumption of 70% and 50% CRPS prevalence. Again, no raw data was provided to reproduce these results. The assumption for this high prevalence of CRPS to calculate positive and negative predictive value is not supported.

In summary, after reviewing the above articles, it was not possible to reproduce the reported sensitivity, specificity, positive and negative predictive values based on the data provided in the articles. The assumption of 70% and 50% prevalence of CRPS is not supported in the literature.[5, 6] Attempts to contact Drs. Harden and Bruehl to clarify the data reported were not successful.

Currently there is no gold standard testing for CRPS. Without this information, the true positive diagnosis of CRPS and the calculation of sensitivity cannot be determined. Similarly, without the true positive, specificity, positive predictive value, negative predictive value cannot be calculated based on the information provided in these articles.

Section 3 References:

1. Galer BS, Bruehl S, Harden RN. IASP diagnostic criteria for complex regional pain syndrome: A preliminary empirical validation study. Clin J Pain. 1998;14: 48 – 54.

2. Harden RN, Bruehl S, Galer BS, Saltz S, Bertram M, Backonja M. Complex regional pain syndrome: are the IASP diagnostic criteria valid and sufficiently comprehensive? Pain. 1999; 83:211–219

3. Bruehl S, Harden RN, Galer BS, Saltz S, Bertram M, Backonja M.External validation of IASP diagnostic criteria for complex regional pain syndrome and propose research diagnostic criteria. Pain.1999; 81: 147–154.

4. Harden RN, Bruehl S, Perez R, Birklein F, Marinus J, Maihofner C.Validation of propose diagnostic criteria (the "Budapest criteria") for complex regional pain syndrome. Pain. 2010;150: 268–274.

5. de Mos M, de Bruijn AG, Huygen FJ, Dieleman JP, Stricker BH, Sturkenboom MC. The incidence of complex regional pain syndrome: a population based study. Pain.2007;129:12-20.

6. Sandroni P, Benrud-Larson LM, McClelland RL, Low PA. Complex regional pain syndrome type 1: incidence and prevalence in Olmsted County, a population based study. Pain. 2003;103:199-207.

Section 4

Review of the
Pathophysiological Theories

There are as many problems associated with the diagnosis of CRPS Type I and CRPS Type II because there are many theories for the etiology or pathogenesis of CRPS.

The author A.T. Borchers and colleagues in an article in *Autoimmunity Review* 2014 entitled "Complex Regional Pain Syndrome: A Comprehensive and Critical Review" [10] stated the problem quite clearly. They stated, "Complex Regional Pain Syndrome (CRPS) is a term used to describe a variety of disorders characterized by spontaneous or stimulus-induced pain that is disproportional to the inciting event, and is accompanied by a myriad of autonomic and motor disturbances in highly variable combinations. There are no standards which can be applied to the diagnosis and which will fulfill definitions of evidence based medicine. Indeed, there are almost as many diagnostic criteria as there are names to this disorder. The umbrella term CRPS has been subdivided into Type I and Type II. CRPS Type I is intended to encompass reflux sympathized dystrophy and similar disorders without nerve injury; while CRPS Type II occurs after damage to a peripheral nerve."

As an introduction to the numerous theories about the pathophysiology of CRPS the authors note, "There are numerous etiological pathophysiological events that have been incriminated with the development of CRPS, including inflammation, autoimmune responses, abnormal cytokine production, sympathetic dysentery disorders, altered blood flow and central cortical reorganization." The authors also point out the problem when they state, "However, the number of studies that have included appropriate controls and have sufficient numbers of patients to allow statistical analysis with appropriate power calculations is vanishingly small."

To quote the authors further, they state, "Complex regional pain syndrome (CRPS) is a term coined by the International Association on the Study of Pain (IASP), to describe disorders characterized by spontaneous or stimulus-induced pain that is disproportionate to the inciting event and accompanied by a variety of autonomic and motor disturbances in highly variable combinations. *CRPS is a syndrome steeped in confusion and often inaccuracy.*"

In addition to that, there is considerable confusion whether the authors are considering CRPS Type I versus CRPS Type II. Some authors appear to be studying and referring to Reflex Sympathetic Dystrophy (RSD). RSD and CRPS are not the same thing. CRPS was deliberately created in a fashion that results in it being different from RSD. Therefore, the theories on pathogenesis are somewhat difficult to distinguish as to whether they are discussing RSD and/or CRPS, and then whether CRPS Type I or CRPS Type II is being discussed.

The authors also note another confusing problem when they state, "Approximately 80 different names for such disorders can be found in the English literature alone, more than 100 in other languages, reflecting the precipitating event, the predominant symptoms, the specialty and country of origin of the treating physician, or the presumed pathogenic mechanism. The most common designations include Sudek's atrophy (or dystrophy), Algodystrophy, Algoneurodystrophy and Reflex neurovascular dystrophy." Also, Beerthuzen[5] in *Pain* 2009 states "There are approximately 72 names for CRPS described in the literature..." Then there is the problem of what appears to be various subtypes in the categories of CRPS Type I. As noted by O'Connell et al,[48] "The heterogenicity in the constellation of signs and symptoms in individual patients classified as CRPS Type I and a great variability in the response to the specific treatments at the very least suggest the existence of a distinct subgroups within different underlying pathophysiological mechanisms."

Borchers et al., recognize the difficulty in studying the pathophysiology of CRPS. They state, "There are almost as many diagnostic criteria as there were names. The resulting patient heterogeneity makes it impossible to compare the results or studies that attempted to elucidate pathophysiological mechanisms or to assess treatment outcomes."[10]

In terms of the patient's heterogeneity, and in terms of variation, it is difficult to determine which criteria are being used in some articles. One frequently does not know which of the specific criteria, (IASP, Bruehl, Veldman) are used to diagnose the entity. This makes any interpretation of the pathogenesis of CRPS suspect, i.e. any discussions of the pathogenesis of CRPS should be taken and interpreted with caution.

In the literature there appear to be several subtypes of the pediatric CRPS Type I. It has been suggested that pediatric CRPS Type I constitutes another subgroup in children and adolescents. In pediatric CRPS, the lower limb is most frequently affected. The limb is more often blue and colder than the healthy side and frequently shows hypo perfusion on three-phase bone scintigraphy. While primary CRPS is a poor prognosticator in adults, the majority of pediatric patients diagnosed with CRPS appear to achieve improvement or central resolution, mainly with physical therapy and cognitive behavior interventions.

Contrastingly, adults, in general, have more involvement with the upper extremities. In adults, the upper extremity is initially red and warmer than the healthy side, and only later, may become cold and bluish. This supposedly indicates hyper perfusion. In addition, RSD/CRPS findings appear to remain persistent despite therapy in the adult population. This raises the question whether pediatric CRPS is a subgroup of the same disorder as in adults or a different entity entirely. This adds considerable difficulty and controversy as to the existence of a single pathogenesis responsible for the different subtypes of CRPS. The confusion and multiple theories regarding the pathogenesis is pointed out by Fukushima, Fernanda, et al.[26]

> "The pathophysiology of CRPS is multifaceted and remains incompletely understood. Several lines of evidence point toward disturbances involving abnormal response to tissue injury, peripheral and central pain sensitization processes, neurogenic inflammation, endothelial dysfunction, disturbed sympathetic-afferent coupling, hyperalgesia priming, somatosensory cortical reorganization, genetic predisposition, and even some degree of autoimmunity."

One has to question how a single pathogenesis can be incriminated with such an abundance of theories.

Variance in clinically different stages of the syndrome and clinical subtypes has been described throughout the literature. The current IASP diagnostic criteria make it a distinction between two general subtypes of CRPS: Type I (RSD) and Type II (Causalgia).

In addition to these two diagnostic categories of CRPS by IASP criteria, there appears to be, in review of the literature, a broadly held opinion that CRPS develops through distinct sequential changes each characterized by different pattern of signs and symptoms. Leading one to ask, "How can one identify a single pathogenetic factor?"

It appears that the most authors take the description by Bonica.[9] In Bonica's description, the early acute stage of CRPS is defined as Stage 1 and is thought to consist primarily of pain/sensory dysfunction (hyperalgesia or allodynia), signs of vasomotor dysfunction, and prominent edema. Stage 2 is known as the "dystrophic stage" and is proposed to evolve 3-6 months after onset and is characterized by more severe pain/sensory dysfunction, vasomotor dysfunction, and development of motor/trophic changes. With three entirely different stages hypothesized, it is difficult to identify a single or even multiple pathophysiologic factors that one can incriminate for the different stages.

Harden[32] points out in 2006, "Although there have been only limited empirical tests of this hypothesized statement of CRPS, the concept is infrequently accepted as fact in the CRPS literature. Harden and colleagues[32] derive three homogenous CRPS patient subgroups based on similar signs/symptom pattern. They note the CRPS subgroups do not differ significantly regarding pain duration; however, the derived subgroups are consistent and suggest that there are three possible CRPS subtypes. The three sub-types are defined as:

1) A relatively limited syndrome where vasomotor signs predominate.

2) A relatively limited syndrome with neuropathic pain/sensory abnormalities predominating.

3) A florid CRPS syndrome similar to "classic RSD" descriptions.

The authors feel that this is consistent while limited previous works argues against three sequential stages of CRPS. The authors suggested a difference between clinical presentation between subgroups I and II might reflect the different diagnosis of CRPS Type I and CRPS Type II, respectively.

Not only is CRPS divided into sub-types, there is a significant heterogeneity of symptoms of patients with CRPS. Harden and colleagues reviewed a large number of patients meeting IASP criteria for CRPS and described the typical symptom pattern. They described spontaneous burning or stinging. However, burning pain is quite common in non-CRPS neuropathic pain conditions and this leads us to question the diagnostic utility of the symptom. They mention hyperesthesia in response to typical mechanical stimuli, for example, clothing resting on affected part of the body. Additionally, patients may relate extreme sensitivity to temperature changes induced by environmental changes or bathing. The authors also note a number of other symptoms common to CRPS patients. The authors point out these criteria of IASP lack sufficient specificity for an autoimmune identity.

In a 2010 review based on current literature, the authors analyzed the epidemiology, etiology, pathophysiology, diagnosis and therapy of CRPS.[40] CRPS consists of symptoms including autonomic (disturbances of skin temperature, color, presence of sweating abnormalities, sensory, pain and hyperalgesia) as well as and motor disturbances (tremor, dystonia). Diagnosis is made is based on clinical signs. Several pathophysiological concepts have been posed to explain the concepts of symptoms of CRPS. The authors document that several pathophysiological concepts have been proposed to explain the complex symptoms of CRPS including: facilitated neurogenic inflammation, pathologic and patho/afferent coupling, and neuroplastic changes within the CNS. Also postulated is that genetic factors may predispose for CRPS. The authors, however, concede, *"The pathophysiological pain syndrome is still controversial."* They note "a growing evidence for an 'inflammatory' as well as 'sympathetic' pathogenesis."

Maihöfner and colleagues in 2010[40] discussed new pathophysiological concepts and therapies stating, "The diagnosis of CRPS is mainly made clinically. There are different diagnostic criteria sets that are currently available. *In the absence of a biomarker, a gold standard for the external validation is still lacking."*

Taha and colleagues[66] noted in 2012, "The precise cause of CRPS remains unclear, and current treatments are not effective in many patients. The mechanism underlying CRPS may differ across patients and even with a single patient over time." Taha and colleagues also state, "The diagnostic criteria are not yet optimal or even standardized. There is no simple, objective, non-evasive marker for monitoring disease activity or the effects of treatment. The present diagnostic criteria CRPS Type I and CRPS Type II depends solely on taking meticulous history and conducting a careful physical examination. *There are no specifics tests (or Gold Standards) to confirm the diagnosis."* The authors also note significantly *"There is no single pathophysiological mechanism that can explain the diversity and heterogeneity of the symptoms."*

At the National Institutes of Health State-of-the-Science Meeting on CRPS held in December 2001[4] it was concluded that the existing research on the mechanism of human CRPS is inadequate. They note it failed to capture the adequate and complex nature observed clinically in patients. It is not clear why CRPS develops in some patients but not in others, despite similar initiating events. No clear predisposing factors have been identified. Again, confirmation that there is no single pathophysiological mechanism to explain the diverse and varying forms of CRPS and the diversity of diagnostic criteria between Veldman, IASP, Budapest IASP and Bruehl criteria.

An article selected for anesthesiologist CME program[11] made the assumption that CRPS is a neuropathic pain disorder with significant autonomic features. The authors express the opinion that research in the past decade substantially increased knowledge, indicating that pathophysiological mechanisms may be *multifactorial*. The authors note, "Relative contribution to the mechanism underlying CRPS may differ across patients and even with a patient over time, particular in transition from (warm CRPS) (Acute) and (Cold CRPS) and

(Chronic)." The authors make the statement the CRPS is the current diagnostic label for the syndrome historically referred to as Reflex Sympathetic Dystrophy.

It is somewhat confusing in trying to distinguish when the authors are speaking of CRPS Type I and/or CRPS Type II. Clearly CRPS Type I, RSD and CRPS Type II are different entities. The authors go on to state, "Despite this traditional diagnostic distinction, signs and symptoms of the two CRPS subtypes are similar and there is no evidence that they differ in terms of pathophysiological mechanisms or treatment responses." CRPS Type I and CRPS Type II appear equated, but yet differ significantly in terms of pathophysiological mechanism and initiation of injury.) Taha and colleagues note, "It has become increasingly accepted that there are multiple mechanisms involved. There is some evidence that subtypes of CRPS may exist, reflecting differing relative contributions of multiple underlying mechanisms."

Forouzanfar and colleagues[25] reviewed randomized controlled trials of treatments commonly used in therapeutic interventions in CRPS. They include sympathetic blocks, radical scavenging, prednisone administration, acupuncture and manual lymph draining. The authors concluded that there was limited evidence for the efficacy of any of these interventions. The authors acknowledged that CRPS is a multifactorial disorder requiring multi-disciplinary treatment. "Current treatment approaches also include cognitive behavioral therapies such relaxation training and replacing catastrophizing cognitions with adaptive cognitions."

PSYCHOLOGICAL

As Borchers and colleagues[10] expressed, "Since the severity and duration of signs and symptoms of CRPS is disproportionate to the inciting event, or such event is even absent, it is often thought that CRPS is of hysterical or psychogenic origin or that psychological factors contribute to its development." They further note, "There are a variety of behaviors in CRPS patients that only allow the conclusion that their symptoms are psychogenic."

The authors refer to the article by Verdugo, R. J and colleagues[75]. The aim of the study by Verdugo and his associates was to try to determine the pathophysiological basis for neuropathic hyperalgesias. The authors studied neurological and neurophysiological evaluations of 132 consecutive hyperalgesic patients. Two discrete entities emerge: Regional pain syndrome (CRPS II and I) respectively. The classic group (34.9%) consisted of sensory motor patterns in a specific nerve root distribution with document nerve fiber dysfunction. The atypical group which consisted of 65.1% demonstrated weakness with interrupted effort, non-anatomical hypoesthesia and hyperalgesia; hypoesthesia reversed by placebo, or typical abnormal movements and physiological normality of motor and sensory pathways.

The authors noted, "In one group, anatomical, physiological, and pathological analysis of the nervous system predicted clinical feature, prognosis, and response to management. The other group departs from anatomic principal. In the 2nd group, symptoms often paradoxically worsen in time, rather that improve with natural repair, become refractory to all therapeutic measures; and when tested through objective neurophysiological methods, the motor and sensory function were normal, even with voluntary movement and reported sensation may appear defective or centrally."

The authors summarize their findings and noted the group of classic (CRPS Type II) patients exhibited a coherent positive sensory motor pattern. Any variance was restricted to anatomic distribution and spinal root and equivalence of peripheral nerve pathology, and was documented objectively through neurological examination and physiological tests. On the other hand, the authors noted that the patients with atypical CRPS Type I group (65.2%) departed from the laws of anatomy and physiology.

Verdugo and colleagues[73] demonstrated that CRPS includes cases with somatoform disorder with overlap of conversion and factitious disorder. They noted that in patients with what the authors classified as chronic "neuropathic" pain were subjected to clinical and laboratory investigations, including placebo of controlled local anesthetic block. Patients that displayed profound regional continuous hypoesthesia and pain entered a study through either one of two criteria: (a) reversal of hypoesthesia after diagnostic block and (b) nerve injury as a cause of hypoesthesia and pain.

Two groups emerge: (1) Patients with profound hypoesthesia reversed by block but without neuropathy and (2) Patients with hypoesthesia that did not reverse and had a neuropathy. No patient with a true neuropathy was found whose cutaneous hypoesthesia improved with block. Spontaneous pain was relieved with placebo in 2/3 of the patients in group 1 and approximately ½ in group 2.

The group 1 patients expressed improved hypoesthesia in response to block and no nerve injury as a cause of sensory dysfunction. Group 2 patients with hypoesthesia, did not improve with placebo and all had a known neuropathy as a cause of their problem.

In conclusion, the authors noted, "Such reversal of hypoesthesia is due to placebo effect, acting on a psychogenic symptom because: (a) 27 out of 27 patients in whom the reversal occurred had absence of nerve disease behind the 'neuropathic' symptoms, (b) 26 out of 27 patients whose hypoesthesias was not anatomical, (c)16-27 patients had other sensory-motor signs that could not be explained as a result of an organic pathology, (give way weakness and punctual denial of hypoesthesia), and (d) the phenomenon was not found in patients with organic neuropathy." The authors noted that in these patients, 24 out of 27 in a series, there is no demonstrable structural based nerve dysfunction. They noted the clinical picture was atypical for peripheral neuropathic damage, "All these patients display evidence of dysfunction of pseudoneurological, psychogenic origin."

The author further noted, "The presence of these neurological phenomena by themselves qualifies the clinical picture of these patients that specifically were diagnosed as 'psychogenic regional pain' or 'pseudo neuropathy' a psychological mediated condition ostensibly due to somatization regardless of whether or not a separate diagnosis is attained through psychiatric criteria." The authors submit the fact that the reversal of hypoesthesia by placebo or lidocaine injection constitutes strong criteria for psychogenicity in patients with similarly neuropathic chronic pains and should be tested routinely in atypical cases (CRPS Type I).

There are cases of somatoform disorders associated with CRPS, some with overlap of conversion and fictitious disorders. Taskaynatan, et al.[67] studied 7 patients with a previous diagnosis of RSD made in the military service. At psychological examination and MMPI, anxiety disorders, and/or depression and conversion disorder was diagnosed in 4 of these. The authors described factitious disorders characterized by the intentional production or claiming physical or psychological symptoms in the presence of the need to assume a sick role. The authors report 7 cases of factitious disorder previously diagnosed with RSD in the military service. The authors note "When the mind/body relationship becomes unbalanced to the point of a disease state, the psyche can manifest several well described disorders such as somatization disorder, conversion disorder, psychogenic pain disorder and factitious disorder."

Two examples of psychogenic origin of CRPS Type I or RSD are in articles by Rodriquez- Marino, et al.[56] and Chevalier Xavier, et al.[16], both reporting incidences of Munchausen Syndrome, simulating RSD.

In an attempt to determine whether CRPS Type I patients were psychologically different from other chronic pain patients, with particular attention to personality pathology, Monti[44] found a high incidence of personality pathology in both groups of CRPS patients and chronic pain patients. Statistical analysis reveal both groups to have a significant amount of major psychiatric comorbidities. In an attempt to determine whether or not CRPS patients were psychologically different or "sicker" than other chronic pain patients in terms of personality pathology, a group of CRPS patients were evaluated and compared to another comparable group of chronic pain patients (disk-related radiculopathy aka DRR). Overall, the authors did not find a significant psychiatric difference between CRPS patients and disk-related radiculopathy (DRR) patients. This brings up the question whether the psychiatric morbidity is a cause of the disease, or if it is a personality dysfunction among chronic pain patients. It is suggested that personality patterns associated with marginal adaptive coping styles decompensate under the stress of injury, disability and pain, resulting in an expression of personality disorder. The question becomes then, which comes first, the chicken or the egg.

Another study investigated the role of psychological factors in the development of CRPS Type I following the fracture of the distal radius.[21] All patients were treated by closed reduction and cast immobilization. The risk of CRPS type I was significantly increased in patients with high trait anxiety scores (P=0.38). The results show that after the fracture of the distal radius and casting immobilization, patients who had an anxious personality had a higher risk of developing CRPS Type I.

The authors also point out, however, that some of the studies report CRPS Type I is a chronic pain condition "and behavioral and intramuscular changes can be due to chronic pain. Therefore psychological abnormalities observed in CRPS Type I patients may be the result, not the cause ." However they note that all the studies mentioned previously with retrospective and psychological features were examined in late phase patients. They question, "why some patients develop CRPS Type I and others do not after almost the same trauma and is still being investigated but is as of yet unsolved."

Further complicating the fact of psychological factors playing a role in CRPS is that some cases report a relationship of conversion neurosis and CRPS Type I[51].

On the other hand Monti[44] suggests that the psychological factors develop in the course of CRPS Type I rather than being the underlying factor, making the suggestion that the long life of CRPS results in a change in the psychological make-up of the person suffering.

Some evidence of controversy is that Harden[33] and colleagues found that higher levels of anxiety prior to surgery were associated with the prevalence of CRPS Type I at the one-month follow up. The presence of anxiety at the baseline did not predict the presence of CRPS at the 3 and 6-month follow up. "Life events" have been considered in the pathogenesis of CRPS Type I[28] defining these people as experiencing more "stressful life events" then the controls.

In studying these reviews Borchers[10] discussed the 2 main results most reviewed. "First, most prospective studies found no relation of the diagnosis of CRPS Type I and depression, anxiety, neuroticism, hostility/anger or extraversion/introversion. Second, the results of retrospective/cross section studies seem to yield contradictive results regarding psychological problems in patients with CRPS Type I. The majority of the studies found no association with psychological factors in CRPS Type I."

For life events[28], the evidence seemed to indicate a relationship with the development of CRPS Type I. They noted that life events could lead to CRPS Type I, "because repeatedly triggered sympathetic system develops an altered catecholamine response resulting in prolonged increase of autonomic arousal."

Beerthuizen and colleagues disagree with the psychological aspect in the etiology of CRPS. They note that the pathophysiology of CRPS is still a matter of debate and psychological factors have been suggested to play role, although the influence is unclear.[5] The purpose of this study was to investigate the evidence of psychological factors on the onset and management of CRPS Type I in adults. This constituted a systematic review of articles selected using Cochran PubMed Line Psych Info and Cinahi since 1980 and 31 articles were identified. Literature reviewed by the authors identified no relationship between CRPS Type I and severe psychological factors. Only "life events" seem to be associated with CRPS Type I. The patients who experienced more "life events" appeared to have a greater chance of developing CRPS Type I.

In conclusion the authors state, "No firm conclusion can be drawn from the literature on this association between psychological factors and the maintenance CRPS. This review did not identify any direct relationship between psychological factors and the development of CRPS Type I, with the possible exception of life events."

DYSTONIA OR ABNORMAL MOVEMENTS

Abnormal movements, frequently classified as dystonia, are another example of the controversy regarding the pathogenesis or objective determinants in CRPS. The literature indicates that the incidence of movement disorders is significantly different in CRPS Type I and CRPS Type II; however, the results are highly contradictory. One series, (Verdugo[74]) notes that abnormal movements or dystonia are seen exclusively only in patients with CRPS Type I. No movement disorders were found in the group with CRPS Type II. However, conversely, other data suggests that movement disorders are significantly higher in patients with CRPS Type II compared with those who have CRPS Type I.[6]

Campero[13] used microneurography to confirm normal C-fiber reactivity in all 13 patients with CRPS Type I, whereas abnormal discharges of suspected C-fibers were not observable in 6 out of 11 patients with CRPS Type II.

Verdugo[74] noted that some movement disorders such as muscle spasm, myoclonus and dystonia are rare in some cohorts, but more frequent in others. Abnormal movements (dystonia, spasms, irregular jerks/ and postural tremors) occurred in 58 of the 379 patients with CRPS Type I but none of the 379 patients with CRPS Type II in Verdugo and Ochoa's study. Birklein[6], with marked contrast, found the combined frequency of myoclonic jerks and dystonia muscle contractions were significantly higher in patients with Type II compared Type I, i.e., 48% versus 27%. Incidentally, there are few descriptions of movement disorders in pediatric CRPS.

This is just an example of the controversy regarding CRPS. The dystonia and myoclonus associated with CRPS, whether psychogenic or not, remains controversial and a subject of intense debate. As long as this discrepancy occurs a resolution is unlikely. It is significant, however, that there are reports of disease resolution with psychiatric counseling and reassurance. Also, patients are demonstrated to show significant improvement with multidisciplinary patient treatment, consisting of cognitive behavioral therapy, occupational therapy and psychotherapy. This would suggest that the dystonia and myoclonus are psychiatric disorders in some CRPS patients.[74]

Another study of CRPS patients with dystonia, demonstrated similar scores for somatoform disassociation as the patients with conversion disorder and significantly higher scores compared with patients with affective disorder.[61] Shiri[64] saw impressive similarities in psychological profiles obtained in MMPI-1 of patients with CRPS I and other patients with conversion disorder including a marked frequency of AXIS I disorders.

In the study by Verdugo[74], between August 1990 and September 1998, patients with diagnostic criteria for CRPS (Type I or Type II) with accompanying abnormal movements, were entered into a prospective study. The patients exhibited various combinations of dystonic spasms, postural action tremor, and irregular jerks and in one case, actual choreiform movements. Only patients with CRPS Type I displayed abnormal movements. The authors noted that in addition to an absence of evidence of structured nerve, spinal cord or intracranial damage, all CRPS Type I patients with abnormal movements, typically exhibited pseudoneurological (normally organic) signs. In some cases malingering was documented by secret surveillance. The authors felt that this confirmed significant differences between CRPS Type I and CRPS Type II, the abnormal movements occurring only in CRPS Type I. They felt that these were "consistently a somatoform or malingering origin, signaling an underlying psychoneurological disorder responsible for the entire CRPS profile." The authors conclude that abnormal movements in CRPS Type I are of malingering or somatoform origin and provide predictive signals of psychogenic dysfunction.

A placebo controlled trial with local anesthetic sympathetic nerve blocks were performed in 37 patients. Spontaneous pain responded significantly to placebo in 43.2% (16 patients). The placebo or lidocaine injections unexpectedly improved cutaneous hypoesthesia in 35% (13 patients). Muscle weakness improved by placebo or lidocaine in 27% of the patients (10 patients). There were three patients with sustained dystonic postural affecting the extremities, the movement disorder completely reversed after placebo injection. The authors noted that no structural peripheral nervous system issue was present in any CRPS patient displaying abnormal movements.

Another study[61]reviewed the clinical features of the 103 patients presenting with fixed dystonia and reported a prospective assessment in investigation of 41 of those patients. The best outcome was seen in the patients who underwent multidisciplinary treatment incorporating reassurance, physical therapy, and occupational therapy, as well as, psychotherapy and psychiatric treatment. The authors noted that while some underlying patients with spinal cord or peripheral neurologic abnormalities need to be excluded, "careful examination offers evidence of somatoform disorder or psychogenic dystonia." The question of whether dystonia or myoclonus associated to CRPS is psychogenic or organic continues to be debated. It is noted that it appears the same data could be interpreted showing either organic or psychogenic origins of CRPS associated with movement disorders and as long as this occurs a resolution is unlikely. However, it is significant that some reports of disease resolution with psychiatric counseling and reassurance, show significant improvement with multidisciplinary patient treatment, consisting of cognitive therapy, occupational therapy and psychotherapy demonstrates that dystonia and myoclonus are psychiatric disorders in some CRPS patients.

In one article[61], CRPS patients with dystonia had similar scores for somatoform disassociation as patients with conversion disorder and significant higher scores compared with patients with affective disorders. Another study revealed significant similarities and psychological profiles obtained by MMPI, i.e. patients with CRPS Type I and patients with conversion disorder and similar finding of AXIS I disorders[64]. Again, this makes the search for the pathophysiology or pathogenesis of CRPS confusing and controversial.

SYMPATHETIC NERVOUS SYSTEM

The characteristics and clinical signs and symptoms of autonomic dysfunction such as edema, changes in skin temperature and color, and hyperhidrosis have been taken to indicate a role of the sympathetic nervous system in the pathophysiology of CRPS.

Much of the support to incriminate the sympathetic nervous system in the development and continued pain in CRPS came from the observation that patients reported pain relief after sympathetic blockade. However, sympathetic blockade was frequently performed without a placebo control and the incidences with placebo responses is high in patients with CRPS.[73] Verdugo was able to cause reversal of hypoesthesia by nerve block or placebo, indicating this was a psychological mediated sign in chronic pseudoneuropathic pain patients. Very few randomized controlled trials have been conducted and results so far indicate that sympathetic blocks are no more effective than placebo.

Pain relief may be reported by patients who show signs of reduced rather than increase in sympathetic activity in the affected limb.[3,25] Sympathetic outflow may be normal even in patients with signs of marked vasoconstriction. The authors also point out there is no correlation between pain relief and the typical clinical signs and symptoms of sympathetic blockade, with respect to time of onset, duration and/or degree. They note that the clinical signs do not allow one to conclusively establish the adequacy of sympathetic blockade.

According to a recent Cochran reviews there is moderate evidence that sympathetic nerve blocks with local anesthetics and IV regional blockade with guanethidine are not effective.[48] Apparently no random controlled trials have been performed to compare sympathetic nerve block and placebo in patients with CRPS. However, it continues to be used at various treatment centers. Clinical signs do not allow one to establish adequacy of sympathetic blockade in the absence of placebo- controlled trials.

Microneurography in 24 patients with CRPS I and II (IASP criteria) found no evidence of receptor activation after sympathetic provocation maneuvers such as mental stress, and changes in intrathoracic pressure.[13]

The literature contains one systematic review of the therapeutic role of local anesthetic sympathetic blockades in patients with CRPS. This review addressed 29 studies in 1,144 patients with CRPS Type I and concludes that critical examination of the studies raises the question of whether sympathetic blockade is of any benefit in CRPS Type I. In their data, less than 1/3 of the patients report temporary relief of pain symptoms following a sympathetic blockade. They also note that it is not clear whether this is due to perhaps placebo effect.[15] The authors' conclusions state, "routine administration of percutaneous sympathetic blockade in patients with CRPS Type I is not useful."

FAMILIAL/GENETIC INFLUENCE ON THE DEVELOPMENT OF CRPS

(Genetic predisposition)

Some observations suggest that genetic determinants may play a role in the predisposition to develop CRPS Type I. Familial cases of CRPS (RSD and Algodystrophy) have been reported and suggest that these patients often experience severe disease, early disease onset, disease recurrences, spreading disease to multiple sites and/or dystonia. In some incidences, affected siblings show identical HLA profiles, however a clear pattern of inheritance cannot be determined as noted in the articles regarding genetic predisposition. Some articles have suggested familial occurrences of Complex Regional Pain Syndrome.[79] Shirani and colleagues reviewed the clinical data on 69 CRPS patients seen between 2000 and 2007, seen at The Interventional Neuralgia Clinic of The Mesa Hospital, Houston. This review identified 4 families with 2 or more members affected with CRPS. There were 6 other patients that indicated a positive family history. The investigators were unable to examine them and did not include them in the report. "This suggests a familial concept of 6% (4 probands in a clinical population of 64 families)." However the authors were unable to determine an inheritance pattern where a single or multiple inheritance patterns exists. The authors were unable to determine with certainty a familial occurrence and noted; "Further studies are needed to determine if DNA profiling or other genetic tools to help to determine the vulnerability to develop CRPS."

A study from the Department of Neurology at University Medical Center Leiden, the Netherlands[19] noted that genetic factors and suggested to play a role in Complex Regional Pain Syndrome (CRPS) but familial occurrences have not been extensively studied. In the study, the authors evaluated familial occurrences in Dutch patients with CRPS.

The families were divided between sCRPS patients (sporadic CRPS) and fCRPS (familial CRPS). Thirty-one CRPS families with two or more affected relatives were identified including two families with 5, four families with 4, eight families with 3, and seventeen families with 2 affected relatives. In comparison with sCRPS patients, fCRPS patients had a younger age at onset, and more often in multiple affected extremities and dystonia. The authors concluded CRPS may occur in a familial form but did not find a clear inheritance pattern. Unfortunately the authors did not distinguish between CRPS Type I and CRPS Type II. The diagnosis of CRPS was made with the IASP criteria. The patients were not examined at the time they had CRPS. Much of this was done by questionnaire.

CENTRAL PROCESSES

Cortical Reorganization

Brain mapping studies have indicated the representation of the CRPS Type I affected hand and the contralateral primary somata central cortex (SI) is significantly smaller compared to the unaffected hand or that of healthy controls and shifted toward a cortical representation of the lip.[39]

Functional MRI (fMRI) during electro stimulation revealed reduced signal strength from SI and SII representation of the stimulated index finger of the affected hand, compared to the healthy hand and noted the extended signal changes correlated with the degree of impairment and tactile discrimination.[54] However, in contrast fMRI during finger tapping with CRPS-affected hand showed significantly larger activation of the vital M1, pace supplementing motor area (Pre-SMA) and SMA proper.

It has been hypothesized that pain can result from a mismatch between intention and sensory (poor perception of vision) feedback and compares this to phantom limb pain after amputation. There is experimental evidence that a sensory-motor mismatch can induce a nominal sensation that ranges from tingling to actual pain in healthy volunteers.[43] The authors postulate that the difficulty that CRPS patients experience when initiating movement and referred sensations are similar to what is seen in amputees and suggest that sensory-motor incongruence may play a role in CRPS patients. The posterior parietal cortex (PPC) plays a central role in integrating visual, tactile, pro-perceptive and vestibular input and copy body information on limb movements in order to construct a body schema (a real time representation of the body in space while monitoring movement). The authors postulate that the cortical reorganization of SI, SII and MI and functional observance in the posterior parietal cortex, contribute to the quantification of pain.

Functional neuroimaging studies have revealed a network of brain regions that are most commonly activated during an experience of acute pain. These include SI, SII, insular, anterior singlets, and prefrontal cortices and less consistently, the thalamus.[68] These regions are referred to as the "pain matrix," but the authors point out that activation of this network is not specific when responding to stimuli, a variety of other reasons are activated that contribute to the pain experience in a context-dependent manner.

The authors note that CRPS Type I resolves more frequently in pediatric compared to adult patients. The pediatric population provided a unique opportunity for comparison between the symptomatic and symptom-free state. They noted that studies involved brushing of an unaffected limb resulted in a large number of activated foci, but brushing the same area after symptomatic resolution of CRPS, produced far fewer activations. After symptom recovery, some of the patients still responded to brushing or cooling of the affected limb, though the stimuli evoked only moderate pain at this time.

The authors suggest, "Although this data suggested pain and possibly central sensation contributed to cortical organization while maladaptive cortical reorganization in turn contributes the maintenance and quantification of pain, both processes may be further enhanced by disturbances in the pain processing pathways."

It should also be noted that in their conclusion, they stated, *"While there are some findings that suggesting that certain of these alterations in central processing may predispose to the development in CRPS, there are as yet no conclusive data on whether reorganization and altered brain processing are the cause or the result of CRPS."* Again it seems as if these authors do not distinguish between CRPS Type I or CRPS Type II and they make the assumption that CRPS is a definable complex for which a Gold Standard Test exists.

CENTRAL PROCESSING

Numerous pathophysiological mechanisms contributing to signs and symptoms of CRPS have been identified. However, a pathophysiological explanation of the disease is still lacking.[7] Briklein and colleagues[7] note that peripheral mechanisms that contribute to CRPS include neurogenic inflammation, peripheral sensitization and sympathetic-afferent coupling. The hypothesis assumes that CRPS is a disease of the central nervous system involving changes in central, sympathetic, somatosensory, and motor symptoms.

During the past years the hypothesis has continued to grow that puts CRPS as a CNS disease. This comes from numerous studies including functional imaging methods. The functional MR-imaging (fMRI), single-photon emission CT (SPECT) and mapping techniques based on electro-encephalography (EEG), magneto-encephalography (MEG), and trans cranial magnetic stimulation (TMS), have been used to study CRPS. Alteration of central somatosensory and motor processing have been detected in patients who are assumed to have CRPS Type I. The authors note, "Many studies provide the evidence for a close relationship between chronic pain and CNS reorganization and somatosensory and motor networks in CRPS."

The authors put forth several hypothetical theories. Two of these theories are:

1) There is persistent nociceptive CNS inputs, probably due to peripheral mechanisms such as neurogenic inflammation, interfere with central networks of tactile perception and motor control, therefore inducing plastic changes in these networks.

2) The disturbance of cortical representation of movement and tactile perception itself promotes pain perception being released and in part cause, in not only consequences of chronic pain in patients with CRPS.

Schwenkreis and colleagues[63] note during the past few years increasing evidence for the hypothesis of CRPS as a CNS disease has come from a number of studies involving functional imaging methods. They note that functional imaging studies have demonstrated reorganization in central somatosensory and motor networks, leading to an altered central processing of tactile and nociceptive stimuli and altered cerebral organization of movement. They opine that many studies provide evidence for the close relationship between chronic pain and CNS reorganization and somatosensory motor in CRPS. The authors hypothesize that persistent nociceptive CNS input is probably due peripheral mechanism, such as neurogenic inflammation and this interferes with central networks of tactile perception of motor control. They postulate this induces plastic changes in these networks. *"Although numerous pathophysiological mechanisms contributing to the clinical signs and symptoms of CRPS have been identified, a pathophysiological explanation of the whole disease is still lacking."*

A study done by supportive research from NIH by The Department of Neurobiology, Harvard Medical School[78] studied the concept of central sensitization. They noted, "Nociceptor inputs can trigger prolonged but reversible increase in the excitability in synaptic efficacy of neurons in central nociceptor pathways, the phenomena of central sensitization. Central sensitization manifests as pain and hypersensitivity, particularly dynamic tactile allodynia, secondary punctate or pressure hyperalgesia, after sensations, and enhanced temporal summation." Clinical cohorts were studied and it was noted that central sensitization is applicable to patients with fibromyalgia, osteoarthritis, musculoskeletal disorders with generalized pain, hypersensitivity, headache, temporal mandibular joint disorder, dental pain, neuropathic pain, visceral pain, and post-surgical pain.

This phenomenon was not specific to CRPS either Type I or Type II. The authors noted, "An important question that still needs to be determined is whether there are individuals with a higher inherited propensity for developing central sensitization than others, and if so, whether this conveys an increased risk in both developing conditions with pain hypersensitivity and their chronification." The author discusses Complex Regional Pain Syndrome and notes that a prominent feature of chronic CRPS Type I is tactile hyperesthesia and pressure hyperesthesia which can be measured as enhanced SI activation by neuromagnetometer. The author discusses multiple syndromes including systemic lupus erythematosus, irritable bowel syndrome, rheumatoid arthritis, premenstrual syndrome and many others listed above. They note, "The overwhelming conclusion from these diverse epidemiological studies is that chronic pain hypersensitivity in the absence of inflammation or nerve damage, results in apparently phenotypically different syndromes depending on the tissues/organs affected." They also note, "Much remains to be learned, particularly which genetic environmental triggers increase the risk of developing central sensitization in particular systems, especially what triggers and sustains the phenomena and what is the response in some individuals for its persistence."

Other authors have noted that recent research suggests that a change in cortical structures can contribute to the pathophysiological of CRPS.[17] A review by Karn provides an overview of studies showing cortical involvement of CRPS including mis-localization of tactile stimuli, changes in size and organization of somatosensory map, changes in motor cortex representation, and body perceptions[17]. Karn notes, "Important questions concerning the precise neuromechanism actually remain unanswered."

There are a number of confusing factors regarding the "central sensitization" theory. Brain imaging studies reveal that following loss of limb, somatosensory cortex may undergo plastic changes (neuroplasticity). The cortical regions with no further afferent input, (e.g. the amputated arm) are "invaded," digesting cortical areas such as a lower face area. One consequence to the central re-mapping phenomena is the experience of referred sensations.[25] A number of studies have sought evidence for referred sensation in CRPS.

While neuroimaging studies have been done and these neuroimaging studies demonstrate the involvement of cortical reorganization in CRPS, the relationship between referred sensation and organization of somatosensory cortex remains to be established.

In fMRI scanning one of the findings was the area of motor cortex contralateral the affected side, was significantly enlarged compared to the ipsilateral prints on the unaffected side. This is a controversial finding because the opposite pattern results were observed in studies of the somatosensory cortex VIZ, in which there was a significant reduction cortical area in CRPS.

The authors noted in conclusion, "Recent research provides empirical support for cortical representation and body perception in CRPS." They also note, "There are limited studies that have evaluated the interventions that target cortical networks." Once again the authors frequently do not distinguish between CRPS Type I and CRPS Type II, nor do they describe as to how the diagnosis was arrived.

However, there is considerable confusion and facts that give one pause for thinking regarding "central sensitization in CRPS." The role of hysteria and immobilization must be taken into consideration.

Immobilization is a common treatment of limb injuries--particularly fractures. As noted in the literature, both adult and pediatric patients with CRPS Type I show a history of immobilization, sometimes without a preceding fracture. This is associated with worsening symptoms. As recognized by the IASP diagnostic criteria, immobilization can produce many of the signs and symptoms of CRPS Type I (including skin temperature changes, pain upon movement, and hyperalgesia nonrestrictive to the single nerve, though not spontaneous pain.)

Borchers et al,[10] looked into immobilization. They noted as recognized by IASP diagnostic criteria, immobilization alone can cause many of the signs and symptoms of CRPS as noted above.

Wrist and ankle fractures are most frequently incriminated as the cause of CRPS Type I[31], although this was a study after distal tibia fracture in rats, the authors compared these changes to those observed after cast immobilization and intact normal rats. Substance P was incriminated as contributing to these factors. The authors postulated that facilitating substance P signal, may also contribute to the vascular and nociceptor abnormalities observed after tibia fracture cast immobilization. The authors felt that immobilization alone can generate a syndrome resembling CRPS in substance P signaling to the vascular and nociceptor changes observed in these models.

Essential to this article is that it noted physical therapy is a cornerstone to CRPS treatment, although there are no controlled clinical data supports. The primary goal with physical therapy serves to mobilize the extremity. Results of this study indicate remobilization can reverse CRPS pathology. It is noted that immobilization alone can cause a CRPS-like syndrome of brief duration. In NK1 receptor antagonist partial reversed spontaneous extravasation, warmth and edema in both models.

This is a study on rats which cannot necessarily be interpreted as indicative of the human condition. This data appears to be more involved with the section of a tail in the rat indicating this would be CRPS Type II. Additionally, the authors noted a similar substance of nociceptor changes observe in sciatic section of CRPS Type II rat model.

Further confusion to the concept of brain sensitization has been provided by Ochoa.[50] Dr. Ochoa noted that frontal images of the brain in patients diagnosed hysterical (motor and sensory) dysfunction and pain, revealed intromission of limbic circuit activation during impaired motor and sensory tasks. Studies with positron emission tomography (PET) scan showed hysterical paralysis to the areas of brain activation with attempting to move the paralyzed extremity and include the pre-motor area. Instead, activation of orbital-frontal and singlet cortex was observed.

As to the functional MRI, other studies[42,76] are pertinent. Vuilleumier describes "reduction of regional cerebral blood flow in the contralateral thalamus and suggests that hysterical conversion deficits may include a functional disorder and striatothalamocortical circuits controlling central motor function and voluntary motor behavior." Studies in patients with chronic atypical neuropathic pain "with predominant affective component" also show abnormal cortical activation in response to painful stimulation, particularly in anterior singlet and prefrontal cortex.

Mailis-Gagnom[41] reported abnormal forebrain and limbic activation in patients with intractable pain in the diagnosis of conversion disorder.

In summary, as noted in the lead article by Borchers[10] and other literature, the pathophysiology of CRPS Type I is poorly understood as reflective in the wide-range of explanatory theories, including: an unregulated sympathetic nervous system[77], an exaggerated neurogenic inflammation of the limb[22,77], a genetic predisposition[72], and immobilization of the limb.[22,30] In addition to these explanations, it was suggested that "psychologically peculiar" patterns have an increased risk of developing CRPS.[71]

One must consider there are approximately 72 names for CRPS described in the literature. Also, frequently the literature does not clearly distinguish between

CRPS Type I and CRPS Type II. Another complicating factor is that there are various criteria for diagnosing CRPS Type I, including IASP, the Bruehl, the Veldman, the Adkins and the Budapest criteria. This makes it impossible for one to determine any significant pathogenesis or determine the pathophysiology of either CRPS Type I or CRPS Type II. As Borchers[10] noted, "There are almost as many diagnosis criteria for Complex Regional Pain Syndrome as there are names for the disorder". He further notes, "It has been shown that CRPS Type I can mean bone or common nerve compression, entrapment, dysfunctional posture, somatoform disorder, self-inflicted or factitious or malingering. These are almost all part of the differential diagnosis but obviously are not always recognized by many treating physicians." This clearly indicates that CPRS is simply a "catch all" and therefore should not be considered a valid diagnostic end point. Therefore, consideration of CRPS Type I and CRPS Type II should be considered an indication for an urgent need for extensive exploration of the differential diagnosis.

As Borchers[10] points out, "What is even more peculiar than explicit exclusion of the diagnosis of CRPS by the existence of other conditions that would otherwise account for the degree of pain and dysfunction, is the invention of a CRPS-NOS (not otherwise specified) category by Budapest consensus panel. This category is intended for patients who partially (partially is not even defined) fulfill the diagnostic criteria but whose symptoms are 'not able to be explained by any other condition'. What could better illustrate that CRPS is a default label rather than a diagnosis."

Borchers and colleagues in their "take home messages" clearly summarize the heterogeneity and difficulties in seeking the pathophysiology of CRPS. Their take home messages are:

- Complex Regional Pain Syndrome is a poorly defined termed used to describe the variety of disorders characterized by pain disproportionate to inciting event.

- There are almost as many diagnostic criteria for Complex Regional Pain Syndrome as there are names for the disorder.

- Numerous etiological pathophysiological events have been incriminated including inflammatory, autoimmunity, neurological disorders, altered blood blow and central cortical reorganization. However, the number of studies involved most often have insufficient patients and lack controls.

- Future research should allow more vigorous standards to allow better understanding of Complex Regional Pain Syndrome including what it is, if *it is,* and when it is.

It is also noted by Schwenkreis[63], "Although numerous pathophysiological mechanisms contribute to clinical signs and symptoms of CRPS have been identified, a pathophysiological explanation of the whole disease is still lacking."

Section 4 References

1.   Albrecht, P. J., "Pathological alterations of cutaneous innervation and vasculature in affected limbs from patients with complex regional pain syndrome." *Pain* 2006,120:244-266

2.   Alexander, Guillermo M., et. al., "Changes in plasma cytokines and their soluble receptors in complex regional pain syndrome." *The Journal of Pain*, Vol 13, No 1(January), 2012:pp10-20

3.   Baron, R., et. al., "Causalgia and reflex sympathetic dystrophy: Does the sympathetic nervous system contribute to the generation of pain?" *Muscle Nerve*, 1999; 22:678-95

4.   Baron, R., et. al., National Institutes of Health Workshop: Reflex sympathetic dystrophy/complex regional pain syndrome – state-of-the science. *Anesth Analg* 2002; 95:1812-6

5.   Beerthuizen, A., et. al., "Is there an association between psychological factors and the complex regional pain syndrome type I (CRPS I) in adults? A systematic review. *Pain* 2009; 145:52-9

6.   Birklein, F., et. al., "Neurologic findings in complex regional pain syndrome-analysis of 145 cases", *Acta Neurol Scand*, 2000;101:262-9

7.   Birklein, F., et. al., "Complex regional pain syndrome: How to resolve the complexity?" *Pain* 2001; 94:1-6

8.   Birklein, Frank, "Complex regional pain syndrome", *J Neurol*, 2005:252:131-138, (ENS Teaching Review)

9.   Bonica, J.J., "Causalgia and other reflex sympathetic dystrophies." N:Bonica, JJ, Ed. Management of Pain, 2nd Ed. Philadelphia: Lea & Febiger, 1990-243

10.   Borchers, A. T., M. E. Gershwin, Autoimmunity Reviews 13, 2014, 240-265, "Complex regional pain syndrome: A comprehensive and critical view."

11.   Bruehl, S., "An update on the pathophysiology of complex regional pain syndrome." *Anesthesiology*, 2010;113(3):713-25

12.   Bruehl, Stephen Ph. D., et. al., "Psychological and behavioral aspects of complex regional pain syndrome management." *Clinical Journal of Pain*, Vol 22, No. 5, June 2006, Pages 430-436.

13.   Campero, M., et. al., "A search for activation of C nociceptors by sympathetic fibers in complex regional pain syndrome". *Clin Neurophysiol*, 2010;121:1072-9

14.   Casale, R., et. al., "Sympathetic nerve activity in reflex sympathetic dystrophy with marked skin vasal constriction" *J Auton Nerv Syst*, 1992;41:215-9

15.   Cepeda, M.S., et. al., "Defining therapeutic role of local anesthetic sympathetic blockade in complex regional pain syndrome: A narrative and systematic review", *Clin J Pain*, 2002,18:216-322

16.   Chevalier X, Claudepierre P, Larget-Piet B, et al. Munchausen's syndrome simulating reflex sympathetic dystrophy. J Rheumatol. 1996;23:1111–1112.

17.   C. M. A. (Karn) Swart, et. al., "Cortical changes in complex regional pain syndrome (CRPS)" *European Journal of Pain* 13 (2009) 902-907

18.   de Mos, M., et. al., "Outcome of the complex regional pain syndrome." *Clin J Pain* 2009; 25:590-7

19.   de Rooij, A. M., et. al., "Familial occurrence of complex regional pain syndrome." *Eur J Pain* 2009; 13:171-777

20.   Department of Anesthesia and Medicine, Université de Montréal, Montreal, QC, Canada. Also, Department of Anesthesia, CHUM-Hospital Notre-Dame, Montreal, Canada

21.   Dilek B, et al. "Anxious personality is a risk factor for developing complex regional pain syndrome type I." *Rheumatol Int* 2012; 32:915–20.

22. Disuse, Butler S. and complex regional pain syndrome. In: Harden RN, Baron R, Janig W, eds. Complex Regional Pain Syndrome. Seattle: IASP Press; 2001

23. Edwards, R. R., et. al., "Association of catastrophizing with interleukin-6 responses to acute pain." *Pain* 2008; 140:135-44

24. Eisenberg, E., et. al., "Serum and salivary oxidative analysis in complex regional pain syndrome." *Pain* 2008,38:226-232

25. Forouzanfar, T., et. al., "Treatment of complex regional pain syndrome, type I," Eur J *Pain*, 2002; 6:105-22

26. Fukushima, Fernanda et al, Complex Regional Pain Syndrome, DMJ 2014; 348;g3683, June 25, 2014

27. Gertzen, J.H., et. al., "Reflex sympathetic dystrophy of the upper extremity-A 5.5 year follow-up, Part II, Social life events, general health and changes in occupations", *Acta Orthop Scand Suppl*, 1998;279:19-23

28. Gertzen, J.H., et. al., "Stressful life events and psychological dysfunction in complex regional pain syndrome type I", *Clin J. Pain*, 1998;14:143-7

29. Glerthmühlen, J., et. al., "Sensory signs in complex regional pain syndrome and peripheral nerve injury", *Pain*, 2012;153:7065-74

30. Gugtz, et. al., "Substance P signaling contributes to the vascular and nociceptive abnormalities observed in a tibial fracture rat model of complex regional pain syndrome type I", *Pain*, 2004;108:95-107

31. Guo, T.Z., et. al., "Substance P signaling contributes to the vascular and nociceptive abnormalities observed in tibial fracture rat model of complex regional pain syndrome type I", *Pain*, 2004;108:95-107

32. Harden, R. Norman, M.D. and Stephen P. Bruehl, PhD., "Diagnosis of complex regional pain syndrome. Signs, symptoms, and new empirically derived diagnostic criteria." Clin J Pain, Vol 22, No. 5, June 2006:415-419

33. Harden, R.N., et. al., "Prospective examination of pain related and psychological predictors of CRPS-like phenomena following total knee arthroplasty: A preliminary study." *Pain*, 2003;106:393-400

34. Janig, W., et. al., "Is CRPS I a neuropathic pain syndrome?" *Pain* 2006, 120:227-229

35. Kingery, W.S., et. al., "An NK_1 antagonist can reverse vascular and nociceptive abnormalities in rat model of complex regional pain syndrome Type II", *Pain*, 2003;104:75-84

36. Kohr, D., et. al., "Autoantibodies in complex regional pain syndrome bind to a differentiation-dependent neuronal surface autoantigen." *Pain* 2009, 143:246-251

37. Lewis, J. S., et. al., "Perceptions of the painful body: The relationship between body perception disturbance, pain and tactile discrimination in complex regional pain syndrome." *Eur J Pain*, 2012;16:1320-30

38. Lynch, M.E., "Psychological aspects of reflex sympathetic dystrophy: A review of adult and pediatric literature", Pain, 1992;49:337-47

39. Maihöfner, C., et. al., "Patterns of cortical reorganization in complex regional pain syndrome." *Neurology*, 2003;61:1707-15

40. Maihöfner, C., et. al., "Complex regional pain syndrome: New pathophysiological concepts and therapies." *European Journal of Neurology*, 2010, 17:649-660

41. Mailis-Gagnon A, et al. Altered central somatosensory processing in chronic pain patients with "hysterical" anesthesia. Neurology. 2003;60:1501–7.

42. Marshall JC, et. al. The functional anatomy of a hysterical paralysis. Cognition. 1997;64:B1–8

43. McCabe, C.S., et. al., "Stimulating sensorimotor incongruence in healthy volunteers: Implications for a cortical model of pain", *Rheumatology* (Oxford) 2005;44:509-16

44.   Monti, et. al., "Personality assessment of patients with complex regional pain syndrome type I", *Clin J Pain*, 1998;14:295-303

45.   Moisset, X., et. al., "Brain imaging of neuropathic pain." *Neuroimage* 2007; 37 (suppl 1): S80-8

46.   Morelet A., et. al., "Tonic dystonia: Uncommon complication of reflex sympathetic dystrophy syndrome. A review of five cases." *Joint Bone Spine* 2005; 72:260-2

47.   Naleschinski, Dennis, Baron, Ralf, "Complex regional pain syndrome type I: Neuropathic or not?" *Curr Pain Headache Rep* 2010 14:196-202

48.   O'Connell, N.E., et. al., "Interventions for creating pain and disability in adults with complex regional pain syndrome.", Cochran Data Base System Rev, 2013;4:CD009416

49.   Oakander, A. L., "Evidence of focal small fiber axonal degeneration in complex regional pain syndrome I" *Pain* 2006,120: 235-234

50.   Ochoa, J. L., Verdugo, R. J., "Reflex sympathetic dystrophy. A common clinical avenue for somatoform expression." *Neurol* 1995; 13:351-63

51.   Parsod, E., et. al., "Conversion disorder after implant of a spinal cord stimulator in a patient with complex regional pain syndrome", *Anesth Analg*, 2003; 96: 201-6

52.   Perez, Roberto S., et. al., "Evidence based guidelines for complex regional pain syndrome Type I", *BMC Neurology*, 2010:20:1-14.

53.   Perez, R. S. "Treatment of reflex sympathetic dystrophy (CRPS Type I): A research synthesis of 21 randomized clinical trials" *J Pain Symptom Manage* 2001; 21:511-25

54.   Prager, Joshua P., M.D., "What does the mechanism of spinal cord stimulation tell us about complex regional pain syndrome", *Pain Medicine*, 2010;11:1278-1283

55. Renato J. Verdugo, M.D., et. al., Abnormal movements in complex regional pain syndrome: Assessment of the nature", *Muscle and Nerve*, February 2000, 198-205

56. Rodriguez-Moreno J, Ruiz-Martin JM, Mateo-Soria L, Rozadilla A, Roig-Escofet D. Munchausen's syndrome simulating reflex sympathetic dystrophy. Ann Rheum Dis. 1990;49:2010–2.

57. Rommel, O., et. al., "Hemi sensory impairment in patients with complex regional pain syndrome.", *Pain*, 1999;80:95-101

58. Sandroni, P, et. al., complex regional pain syndrome type I: Incidence and prevalence in Olmsted County, a population-based study. *Pain* 2003;103:199–207

59. Sato J., et. al., "Adrenergic excitation of cutaneous pain receptors inducted by peripheral nerve injury." *Science* 1991; 251:1608-10

60. Schott, G. G., "Peripherally-triggered CRPS and dystonia." *Pain* (2007) 203-207 The authors from the National Hospital for Neurology and Neurosurgery, Queen Square, London

61. Schreg, Annette., et. al., "The syndrome of fixed dystonia: An evaluation of 103 patients." *Brain*, 2004;127:2360-72

62. Schwartzman, Robert J., et. al., "Pathophysiology of complex regional pain syndrome." *Expert Rev Neurotherapeutics* 6 (5), 2006:669-81

63. Schwenkreis, et. al., "Functional imaging of central nervous system involved in complex regional pain syndrome", Departments of Neurology and Pain Management, Ruhr-University Bochum Germany. This is in *AJNR Am.*, 30:1279-84, August 2009.

64. Shiri, S., et. al., "Similarities between the psychological profiles of complex regional pain syndrome and conversion disorder patients", *J Clin Psychol Med Settings*, 2003;10:193-9

65. Szein-Berg-Arazi, D., et. al., "A functional and psychological assessment of patients with post-Sudeck's atrophy amputation", *Arch Phys Med Rehabil*, 1993;74:416-8

66. Taha, Rame M.D., et. al. "Update on the pathogenesis of complex regional pain syndrome: role of oxidative stress." *Can J Anaesth* 2012 59:875-881.

67. Taskaynatan MA, Balaban B, Karlidere T, et al. Factitious disorders encountered in patients with the diagnosis of reflex sympathetic dystrophy. Clin Rheumatol. 2005;24:521–526.

68. Tracey, I., et. al., "The cerebral signature for pain perception and its modulation", *Neuron*, 2007;55:377-91

69. Trede, R. D., et. al., "Neuropathic pain: Redefinition and a grading system for clinical and research purposes." *Neurology* 2008, 70:1630-1635

70. Turner, J.A., et. al., "Spinal cord stimulation for chronic low back pain: A systematic literature synthesis", *Neurosurgery*, 1955,37:1088-1095

71. van Houdenhove, B., et. al., "*Idiopathogenesis* of reflex sympathetic dystrophy: A review and biosocial hypothesis", Clang J Pain, 1992 (4):300-6

72. Vaneker, M., et. al., "Genetic factors associated with complex regional pain syndrome I: HLA-DRB and TNF Alpha Promoter Gene Polymorphism.", *Disabl Med*, 2002;2:69-74

73. Verdugo, R. J., et. al., "Reversal of hypoesthesia by nerve block, or placebo: A psychologically mediated sign in chronic pseudoneuropathic pain patients." *J Neurol Neurosurg Psychiatry* 1998; 65:196-203)

74. Verdugo, R.J., Ochoa, J. L., "Abnormal movements in complex regional pain syndrome: Assessment of their nature." *Muscle Nerve*, 2000;23:198-205

75. Verdugo RJ, Bell LA, Campero M, Salvat F, Triplett B, Sonnad J, Ochoa JL. Spectrum of cutaneous hyperalgesias/allodynias in neuropathic pain patients. Acta Neurol Scand. 2004;110:368–76.

76.   Vuilleumier P, Chicherio C, Assal F, Schwartz S, Slosman D, Landis T. Functional neuroanatomical correlates of hysterical sensorimotor loss. Brain. 2001;124:1077–90

77.   Wesner, G., et. al., "Complex regional pain syndrome-Diagnostic mechanisms, CNS involvement in therapy." *Spinal Cord Journal*, 2003;41:61-75

78.   Wolf, Clifford, J., "Central sensitization: Implications for diagnosis and treatment of pain", *Pain*, 152(2011), S2-S15

79.   Shirani P, Jawaid A, Moretti P, Lahijani E, Salamone AR, Schulz PE, Edmondson EA. Can J Neurol Sci. 2010 May;37(3):389-94.

Section 5

The Critical Significance of the Differential Diagnostic Process (Physical)

PHYSICAL CAUSES

INTRODUCTION:

The evaluation of an individual with a painful limb(s) requires a thorough knowledge of the history, review of systems, comorbidities and physical examination, and appropriate laboratory studies of the patient. This section will discuss common causes of painful limbs and address the differential diagnosis in association with the default condition of CRPS.

No pathophysiologic process has been proven for this default condition. No "gold standard" exists to confirm "true positives". The process of differential diagnosis is uncommonly encountered. The 4th IASP criteria, that "no other diagnosis better explains the signs and symptoms"[1] is generally ignored.

Absent a reasonable attempt at ruling out common causes of painful limbs, a diagnosis of CRPS should not be provided. Therefore, an exhaustive differential diagnostic process is warranted prior to concluding the presence of the default condition CRPS 1 or 2.

THE EVALUATION OF HISTORY AND SYMPTOMS:

The initial evaluation of an individual with a painful limb should begin with an extensive clinical history. This should include the date and mechanism of the onset of the complaints, the anatomic distribution, and a description of the manifestation of those complaints (i.e. numbness, tingling, burning, sharp pain, dull ache, color and temperature changes, altered sweat patterns, changes in nail and hair growth, etc.). Involvement of multiple limbs and the distribution in each limb (with attention to symmetry or asymmetry, anatomic vs non-anatomic distribution) should also be documented.

Autonomic symptoms are frequently discussed within a CRPS presentation. These symptoms (Table 1) may reflect systemic involvement and complete evaluation for systemic causes is warranted. Autonomic symptoms can commonly be seen with peripheral neuropathies in association with metabolic or nutritional conditions; such as: diabetes, vitamin/nutritional deficiencies, inherited neurologic abnormalities, alcohol abuse, malignancy, medication effects including drug-drug and drug-disease interaction, renal and/or liver failure and autoimmune/connective tissue disorders[2-4].

Autonomic symptoms can include postural hypotension, cardiac dysrhythmia, impairment of sweat pattern, gastrointestinal motility disorders, edema, nausea, vomiting, constipation, genitourinary dysfunction, and dryness of the eyes or mouth (Table 1).

Historic risk factors associated with the development of a painful limb are noted in Table 2. The review of systems should address these more common conditions. If historic information cues any of the common conditions as potential diagnostic considerations, laboratory evaluation is warranted. An overview of the most common diagnostic considerations regarding the painful limb is provided (Table 3).

DIFFERENTIAL DIAGNOSIS OF PAINFUL LIMB(S) AND PAINFUL PERIPHERAL NEUROPATHY (PPN):

Peripheral neuropathies are a common cause of painful limb complaints. Peripheral neuropathies have been subdivided into causes[5]. Each potential etiology requires historic investigation. Autonomic dysfunction may also be seen and would be easily confused with the described clinical picture of CRPS type 1.

The characterization of neurologic anomalies is important in the evaluation of a painful limb. Peripheral nerves provide sensory, motor and autonomic functions. Pathologic peripheral nerve processes may present as separate or mixed abnormalities. Complaints may be symmetric or asymmetric, and may involve single or multiple limbs. Common medical problems can present as peripheral neuropathies[6]. These risk factors are summarized in Table 2. Common causes will be presented as etiologic categories.

Congenital:

Hereditary sensory/autonomic neuropathy represents a group of conditions of genetic etiology. Motor involvement is not usually seen. A family history may be available. Initial presentation may involve traumatic or burn wounds due to sensory loss. These may heal poorly, with ulcer formation and infection. Examples include Fabry's disease, amyloidosis and porphyria[7].

Fabry's disease is a recessive X-linked disorder and occurs due to lipid metabolizing enzyme deficiency. Symptoms usually begin in childhood and are accompanied by painful hand spasms with burning. Autonomic symptoms such as decrease in sweat patterns, and GI problems associated with dysmotility can be seen.

Amyloid neuropathy occurs when a protein (amyloid) is deposited in peripheral nerves, producing mixed motor/sensory and/or autonomic symptoms. This is often accompanied by multi-system involvement, including renal, hepatic, and cardiac.

Porphyria is a group of rare disorders which can be either inherited or acquired due to exposure to certain drugs (e.g. sulfonamides, barbiturates). Chronic neuropathic pain with autonomic GI complaints can be seen with porphyria.

Toxic Causes:

Toxic exposures to various ingested and/or environmental toxins including alcohol, metals (lead, arsenic, mercury and thallium), organic solvents, certain prescription medications (anti-neoplastics, amiodarone, statins), and certain insecticides are recognized as having neurotoxic impact on peripheral nerves[8] (Table 2).

Chronic alcoholism is a very common cause of limb pain from peripheral neuropathy. Alcoholism can produce a mixed sensory/motor/autonomic neuropathy in up to 66 % of individuals with this condition[9]. A "mixed" appearance may be due to direct toxic effects of alcohol and metabolites and nutritional deficiencies noted in this population, including thiamine deficiency— which is commonly encountered. This nutritional issue may be due to a diminished ability to properly absorb and/or metabolize nutrients such as thiamine. Both sources of PPN may be simultaneously present. The source of alcohol should also be a consideration as "homemade" alcohol can be contaminated with toxic metals such as lead[5,10-13].

Lead induced peripheral neuropathy is usually accompanied by other signs of systemic toxicity, such as CNS involvement, anemia, generalized weakness, myalgia, and encephalopathic symptoms. Generalized motor slowing can be seen on EMG. Toxic peripheral neuropathies can also be seen as a consequence of exposure to mercury, arsenic and thallium[14].

Organophosphate insecticides can produce a sensorimotor peripheral neuropathy which is generally delayed after exposure. Direct cholinergic effects of these compounds can also lead to autonomic symptoms[15,16].

Organic solvents, both aliphatic and aromatic varieties (glues, trichloroethylene, benzene) have been shown to have direct toxic effects on peripheral and central neural tissue[17]. These effects are primarily sensorimotor and may also be accompanied by encephalopathic findings[16].

Pharmacologic:

Pharmaceutical preparations have been found as causes of painful mixed peripheral neuropathies. Common cancer chemotherapeutic agents such as cisplatin, oxaliplatin and vinca alkaloids can produce a mixed sensory and motor neuropathy, due to direct toxic effects on neural tissue. It is noted that significant diminution in the extent of peripheral neuropathies due to cisplatin were achieved with vitamin E pre-treatment[5,9,18-20].

Bortezomid is a chemotherapeutic agent utilized to treat multiple myeloma and certain lymphomas. This medication can produce painful small fiber neuropathic pain, with sensory, motor and autonomic features[21]. Antiviral drugs have been found associated with similar toxic results[22].

Commonly used medications such as amiodarone, allopurinol, colchicine, dapsone, isoniazid, phenytoin, glutethemide, and nitrous oxide have been associated with peripheral neuropathies. Statins have been linked to peripheral neuropathy, even when controlling for co-morbidities[23].

Trauma:

Direct trauma to a peripheral nerve can lead to a PPN. This is commonly seen overlying the medial epicondyle of the elbow (ulnar neuropathy) or knee (peroneal neuropathy)[24]. Such trauma can lead to local acute and/or chronic inflammation and an entrapment may occur. Resultant pain may be identified as "CRPS 2" when a discrete nerve is identified.

Localized cellulitis may also produce a painful limb, as could spasm from local muscle trauma. These conditions should be easily distinguished from other peripheral neuropathic pictures, as they are often acute, with clarifying historic information usually available.

Systemic conditions:

Chronic renal failure may result in peripheral polyneuropathy with autonomic features due to circulating uremic toxins. Diminution of symptoms with dialysis may occur. A similar clinical presentation has been reported among those with liver failure[19]. However, many of these complaints are seen in patients with co-morbid conditions separately associated with PPN (hepatitis, alcoholism) [25,26].

Mononeuritis (or polyneuritis) multiplex is a PPN associated with a number of metabolic and immune mediated conditions including diabetes, vasculitis, rheumatoid arthritis, lupus, sarcoidosis, amyloidosis, cryoglobulinemia, and various infectious etiologies (e.g. leprosy, lyme disease, HIV, hepatitis B and C). If multiple nerve trunks are involved, the term "polyneuritis multiplex" is applied. Complaints reflective of sensory, motor and autonomic involvement may develop slowly or more rapidly, depending on the underlying process. Inflammatory cell infiltration characteristic of the autoimmune conditions can produce pain in symmetric or asymmetric patterns, with EMG studies showing sensory and motor multifocal axonal neuropathies[27-35].

Raynaud's phenomenon may be primary (idiopathic) or a secondary phenomenon seen in association with a variety of connective tissue diseases. It is a vasospastic condition usually of the hands. When it occurs in conjunction with autoimmune, chronic inflammatory or connective tissue diseases, symptoms of autonomic dysfunction may also be seen[2,36].

Cancer has been associated with the occurrence of PPN. This can occur when there is direct involvement of the neural tissues, local or distant metastasis, or with a paraneoplastic syndrome (e.g. small cell lung cancers, bladder cancers, rectal cancers and thymomas).[37] Symptoms may be due to neuronal autoantibodies, chemotherapeutic agents, or both.[2,37]

Amyloidosis can produce a PPN with autonomic features and polyneuropathy[6]. These symptoms are seen in association with light chain immunoglobulins, also associated with multi system involvement.

Sarcoidosis is a chronic inflammatory disease and is associated with the development of small fiber neuropathy (SFN). This produces a mixed sensory/motor and autonomic PPN due to damage to small myelinated and unmyelinated nerve fibers. See further comments below on SFN.

Rheumatologic connective tissue conditions can also produce painful peripheral neuropathies which may be limited to a single extremity. Such conditions include lupus, rheumatoid arthritis, mixed connective tissue disease, Sjögren's syndrome, and scleroderma[30,31,33].

Peripheral neuropathies are common in renal failure, hepatic disease, and pulmonary disease (pulmonary failure). They have been reported to produce neuropathy in half of these populations[5].

Inflammatory bowel disease such as celiac disease, Crohn's disease and ulcerative colitis have also been reported to be associated with painful peripheral neuropathies occurring in up to 30% of this population. This is generally attributed to vitamin B12 absorption deficiencies.[19,38,39] GI symptoms which defy diagnoses may reflect dysautonomia.[40]

Vasculitis has also been reported to result in painful peripheral neuropathies. This includes conditions such as polyarteritis nodosa, microscopic polyangiitis, giant cell arteritis and hypersensitivity vasculitis.[36,41]

Secondary vasculitis from lupus, rheumatoid arthritis, Sjögren's syndrome, sarcoidosis, cytomegalovirus infections, and paraneoplastic syndromes have been reported to produce painful peripheral neuropathies.[36]

Infectious:

Multiple chronic viral conditions such as Hepatitis B and C, HIV, Herpes, Epstein-Barr, and cytomegalovirus infections can lead to PPN[42-44]. The etiology is unclear. Post-herpetic neuralgia is a common example. Other severe viral infections have been associated with mixed peripheral neuropathies and mononeuritis multiplex. Some medications used to treat these viral conditions have also been associated with PPN.[43-47]

Leprosy and Lyme disease is associated with both PPN and mononeuritis multiplex. Diphtheria can produce a late onset demyelinating polyneuropathy. Borreliosis and syphilis can produce a primarily sensory neuropathy.[48-50]

Historic information to evaluate recent infectious processes, including pertussis, diphtheria, tuberculosis, herpes-zoster, unusual rashes or skin lesions, or a history of chronic skin conditions such as psoriasis should be documented. A history of recent travel, especially to tropical areas could be important in the differential diagnostic process.

A history of substance abuse, especially IV drug use should raise suspicion for possible infectious etiologies of PPN.

Endocrine:

Diabetes is a very common cause of PPN, potentially producing mixed sensory, motor, and autonomic symptoms. PPN symptoms may also be seen in patients with only impaired glucose tolerance. Diabetes of variable levels of control has been associated with significant multisystem autonomic neuropathy and rheumatic complaints[51]. A thorough review of systems is encouraged to address this in susceptible patients. Impaired glucose tolerance alone (without clear diagnosis of diabetes) has also been associated with PPN[27,52-55].

Cardiovascular symptoms should be carefully reviewed to include episodes of congestive heart failure, irregular heartbeat, high blood pressure, dizziness, or episodes of syncope. Neurologic symptoms such as diplopia, blurred vision, generalized weakness or fatigue, increasing forgetfulness, visual disturbances of any kind, or dementia /cognitive disturbances should also be reviewed. Such multi-system involvement may be indicative of an autonomic disorder such as diabetic dysautonomia[3,4,56-59].

Hypothyroidism has been associated with PPN. The onset of symptoms can be over the course of years. Thyroid function should be evaluated in the patient with PPN[60,61].

Nutritional and Metabolic:

Obesity is recognized as being associated with nutritional deficiencies. Individuals undergoing gastric bypass surgery are well recognized to present both acutely and remotely with multivitamin and nutritional deficiencies[51,53,62-64]. PPN have also been described in those diagnosed with the "Metabolic Syndrome" of obesity, diabetes and hypertension.[65]

Obese individuals have been reported to have evidence of significant vitamin D deficiencies, anemia, iron deficiency, B12 deficiency and folate deficiency[66]. Those undergoing bariatric surgeries, especially the gastric bypass procedures have been reported to have multivitamin deficiencies involving vitamin B complex, vitamin D, vitamin E, vitamin A, copper, zinc and selenium deficiencies. The occurrence of the peripheral neuropathies in association with obesity and bariatric surgery may be acute (within six weeks of the surgery) or may not occur for more than 10 years after the fact[67,68].

The mechanism of the deficiency centers around malabsorption. Critical absorption portions of the gastrointestinal tract (stomach and duodenum) may be removed from exposure to ingested food (as in the "Roux-en-Y" procedure).In this situation, inadequate vitamin D prevents the absorption of B12 [66,69-71].

The most common vitamin deficiencies involve the B complex (primarily vitamin B1 or thiamine, and vitamin B12). Thiamine deficiency (beriberi) can be seen in absorption states, such as chronic alcoholism, and can produce painful peripheral neuropathies as well as cardiomyopathy. B12 deficiencies, also common in malabsorption states, can lead to pernicious anemia--a sensory ataxia with combined spinal cord degeneration of a subacute nature with spastic paraparesis[40,72].

If gastric bypass surgery has been performed, the date and type of bypass procedure should be documented accompanied by a history of the nature of the weight loss including total weight loss and the duration over which the weight loss occurred. More rapid and higher quantity weight loss is accompanied with more significant nutritional deficiencies and, therefore, a greater likelihood of the establishment or development of a peripheral neuropathy. Some individuals elect to discontinue routine follow-up visits and nutritional supplementation following these procedures. These patients are at greater risk for malnutrition and may present remotely with PPN[66,73].

Malabsorption states seen in obesity and gastric bypass can involve vitamins A, D, E, and K[40]. Sensory loss is noted with vitamin E involving large fibers. Vitamin E deficiency may also lead to ataxia[67,74].

Vitamin D deficiency is common in morbidly obese and individuals who have had bariatric bypass procedures. This may be accompanied by calcium and phosphorus deficiency and may also be linked to hyperparathyroidism. Vitamin D deficiencies have been associated with myopathy and cutaneous hyperalgesia[75].

A history of anemia should also be discussed and the source determined. This recommendation is based on the association of anemia with multiple systemic and nutritional deficiencies and/or toxicities (e.g. lead). A thorough assessment of the cause of the anemia is warranted, especially when present with a PPN.

Small Fiber Neuropathy (SFN)

SFN is often idiopathic, but shares etiology with other painful peripheral neuropathies[76]. It can present as a painful neuropathic process involving sensory, motor, autonomic, or mixed components. Diagnosis is based on quantitative sensory testing (QST), abnormal clinical exam, and skin biopsy showing quantification of somatic intra-epidermal nerve fibers (IENF). The cause is often not found, but, nevertheless, this condition bears consideration in the differential diagnosis of CRPS 1.[77] A suspicion of SFN should be raised in patients with PPN symptoms with limited objective findings and increasing symptoms. SFN may appear in individuals with impaired glucose tolerance.

EXAMINATION OF AN INDIVIDUAL WITH A PAINFUL LIMB:

Following the history and review of systems, all of the patient's medications should be documented with doses and frequency. Over-the-counter, vitamin/mineral and herbal preparations should also be documented as many of these over-the-counter preparations have metabolic impact and potential drug-drug interactions with other ingested pharmaceuticals.

An examination of the extremities should include descriptions of the skin turgor and appearance, evidence of lesions (e.g. psoriasis), temperature, hair growth differences or variations, appearance of the nails, documentation of posttraumatic or postsurgical scars and tattoos. Circumferential measurements should be obtained symmetrically in at least two locations in each extremity and should be documented to address issues of atrophy or swelling/edema. Sensation and motor strength of major muscle groups should be tested. Delineation of altered sensation through fine touch, two-point discrimination, vibration and proprioception should also be documented if there is a concern regarding neuropathic processes, autonomic dysfunction and/or CNS involvement. The distribution of altered perception to fine touch or painful stimulus should be documented to determine if the distribution is anatomic (that is, following a recognized nerve root distribution), or reflective of toxic/metabolic or even a non-physical abnormality (stocking glove distribution).[60]

An individual with a known history of endocrine disorder(s) and a PPN should be the subject of considerable scrutiny. A prior history of hypothyroidism deserves repeat evaluation of the endocrine axis, and EMG should be considered[78]. "Borderline" or controlled diabetes should be assessed with fasting blood sugar, Hgb A1C, and possibly a 2 hour glucose tolerance test, due to the relationship of PPN and dysautonomia with impaired 2 hour glucose tolerance test[78].

The quality, validity, and reliability of electrodiagnostic studies are provider driven. Electro diagnostics in a patient with significant complaints should be tested by a medically trained physician with board certification in Neurology or PM&R, with fellowship training in electro diagnostic testing.

Abdominal tenderness may be an indication to proceed with ultrasonography to assess hepatic or splenic enlargement.

Observations regarding responses to the exam should be documented. "Allodynia" (painful response to non-painful stimulus) and "hyperpathia" (exaggerated painful response to painful stimulus) are subjective, but should be documented for comparison with subsequent exams.

LABORATORY EVALUATION AND DIAGOSTIC STUDIES:

Initial diagnostic studies of an individual with PPN initially should include a complete blood count with differentials and platelets (CBC d/p), metabolic profile to include calcium and phosphorus, blood urea nitrogen and serum creatinine ratio (BUN/CR), electrolytes, fasting blood sugar and glycated hemoglobin (Hg A1C), thyroid function panel and urinalysis. Liver function studies including gamma glutamyl transferase (GGT) should also be performed. An erythrocyte sedimentation rate (ESR) and Vitamin B12 and methylmalonic acid levels should also be drawn. Urinary drug testing to include alcohol is also a consideration[6].

Since metabolic syndrome has been associated with PPN, routine cholesterol and triglyceride testing should be considered.

Routine x-rays of the involved extremities should initially be considered only if a clinical suspicion of trauma or pathologic fracture exists. Comparison views of the uninvolved side may be helpful. Chest x-ray and EKG may also be warranted if there is a suggestive history.

If there has been a history of obesity (BMI greater than 30), a gastric bypass procedure, major GI surgery, or inflammatory bowel disease (Crohn's or ulcerative colitis), then serum levels of vitamins B1, B6, B12, methylmalonic acid, vitamins D, E, and trace minerals (copper, zinc and selenium) should be obtained as all have been linked to painful peripheral mono and polyneuropathies. These levels should be tested even if the patient is taking supplements, as absorption may be diminished due to surgery, underlying malabsorption conditions and/or inflammatory bowel disease[68].

Non-physical issues of psychiatric etiology are noteworthy and subject of the next section of this chapter. It must be noted that such issues will not be uncovered by lab studies, and can often escape detection due to careful masking by patients and/or family members. The patient and/or family members/friends should be questioned pertaining to mental status changes, mood changes or unusual observed behaviors, including problems with cognition, judgment and mentation. Should exhaustive evaluation fail to detect a clear etiology, or if the physician has suspicion of non-physical contributions, a thorough evaluation with psychometric testing should be considered.

Advanced testing is warranted if subjective complaints remain concerning and primary testing unrevealing. Diabetes may be present despite normal fasting blood glucose. A glucose tolerance test should be considered, especially if there are risk factors such as obesity or family history.

If there are significant findings or historic concerns in the extremities, then electro-diagnostic studies should be performed to include electromyography and nerve conduction studies. Consideration for multiple extremity testing to evaluate for neuropathic processes should be considered.

Further advanced testing can include a C-reactive protein, serum protein electrophoresis, venereal disease research laboratory test (VDRL), human immunodeficiency virus (HIV), hepatitis panel, antinuclear antibody test (ANA), and Lyme antibodies. Serum and urine testing for metal toxicity (e.g. lead, mercury) and immunofixation studies could also be performed if there is a concern over demyelinating conditions or myeloma.

If autoimmune conditions are implied by initial test results, further more specific tests pursuing these would be warranted. Such tests could include levels of angiotensin converting enzyme (Sarcoidosis), anti-sulfatide antibodies (autoimmune polyneuropathy), and cerebrospinal fluid analysis for demyelinating conditions. Historic information of hereditary neuropathic processes (Charcot-Marie-Tooth) could be confirmed with genetic testing.

If there remains a suspicion of neurologic abnormalities despite unsuccessful electro diagnostics, a skin biopsy looking for small fiber neuropathy (SFN) may be warranted as this form of pathology will not be detected by standard electro diagnostic studies including EMG and nerve conduction studies.

Due to the complexity and broad scope of the differential diagnostic considerations, a three-tiered approach to the patient with PPN is suggested, first evaluating for more common factors and then widening the scope of the diagnostic processes if simpler testing is not fruitful (Table 4). If evidence points to a suspected etiology (e.g. positive GTT, rheumatoid factor, etc.), then CRPS becomes a remote consideration, and treatments should begin toward known and explainable pathologic processes.

TABLE 1: Common Symptoms of Autonomic Dysfunction: [2,4]

SKIN

- Pallor
- Cyanosis
- Loss of hair
- Thickening of nails
- Discoloration of nails
- Skin mottling/redness
- Thermoregulatory

CARDIOVASCULAR

- Syncope
- Arrhythmias/palpitations
- Unstable blood pressure
- Orthostatic hypotension

GASTROINTESTINAL

- Nausea/vomiting
- Constipation
- Diarrhea
- Abdominal pain
- Gastroparesis
- Bloating

SUDOMOTOR/PUPILLOMOTOR

- Hyperhydrosis (usually hands)
- Dryness of mouth/eyes
- Excessive salivation
- Blurred vision
- Pupillomotor disturbances

GENITOURINARY

- Urinary hesitancy & urgency
- Erectile dysfunction
- Vaginal dryness
- Retrograde ejaculation

TABLE 2:
Historic Factors Creating Physical Risk for Painful Limb

- Family history painful neuropathy/debilitating illness (Lupus, rheumatoid arthritis)
- Cancer
- Obesity
- Gastric bypass surgery of any kind
- Significant abdominal surgery
- Connective tissue disorder
- History of vitamin/nutritional deficiency
- History of HIV, cytomegalovirus, herpes infection
- Anemia
- Diabetes/endocrine disorder
- Substance abuse (alcohol, IV drug use)
- Hepatitis
- Chronic illness requiring medication(s)
- Inflammatory bowel disease (e.g. Crohn's, Ulcerative Colitis)
- History of chronic/significant exposure to neurotoxins (e.g. lead, insecticides, solvents)

TABLE 3: Differential Diagnosis of the Painful Limb: Commonly Encountered Diagnoses

Congenital Causes

- Hereditary sensory/autonomic neuropathies
- Fabry's disease
- Amyloidosis
- Porphyria

Endocrine

- Hypothyroidism
- Diabetes[79, 80]
- Impaired glucose Tolerance

Trauma

- Secondary localized spasm
- Thrombosis
- Entrapment neuropathy
- Cellulitis

Inflammatory

- Acute inflammatory demyelinating neuropathy (Guillain-Barre syndrome)
- Chronic inflammatory demyelinating polyneuropathy
- Inflammatory Bowel Disease (Crohn's Disease, Ulcerative Colitis, Celiac Disease)

Systemic Conditions

- Chronic Renal failure
- Hepatic failure
- Peripheral Vascular dx
- Raynaud's disease
- Vasculitis
- Connective tissue disorders (Rheumatoid arthritis, Lupus, Sjögren's syndrome)
- Cancer (paraneoplastic syndromes, direct neural tissue metastasis, CNS involvement)
- Systemic amyloidosis
- Sarcoidosis (SFN)

Infectious

- Hepatitis B
- Hepatitis C
- HIV
- Epstein - Barr virus
- Herpes Varicella-Zoster
- Herpes Simplex
- Cytomegalovirus
- Lyme disease
- Diphtheria
- Leprosy
- Borreliosis
- Syphilis

Pharmacologic

- Chemotherapy agents (e.g. Cisplatin, Vinca alkaloids)
- Cardiovascular (Amiodarone, Perhexilene)
- Antibiotics (e.g., Isoniazid, Metronidazole, Dapsone)
- Phenytoin
- Etanercept
- Allopurinol
- Triazole (fungicides)
- Chronic steroids

Toxic Causes

- Heavy Metals
- Organic Solvents
- Nitrous oxide
- Organophosphate Insecticides
- Ciguatera toxicity
- Chronic alcoholism

Nutritional/Metabolic Disorders

- Vitamin B1, B6, B12
- Vitamin D (chronic pain syndromes)
- Vitamin E
- Trace Mineral Deficiency (Copper, Zinc, Selenium)
- Hyperlipidemia[79,80]

Other

- Small Fiber Neuropathy (SFN) [79, 80]

TABLE 4a:
A THREE PRONGED APPROACH TO EVALUATION OF THE PAINFUL LIMB

I. **For the patient with NO KNOWN OR IDENTIFIED RISK FACTORS**

A) A THOROUGH HISTORY AND EXAM to include complete review of systems focusing on neurologic, cardiac, gastrointestinal, and musculoskeletal complaints, dysautonomia.

B) Lab studies including fasting blood sugar, bun/creatinine, liver function studies with GGT, CBC, ESR, RA, Vitamin B12 and methylmalonic acid, vitamin D, electrolytes with serum calcium and phosphorus, urinalysis, Hgb A1c, lipid panel, Chest X-ray, and EKG.

C) If there are abdominal complaints and/or tenderness, consider abdominal ultrasound and/or CT looking for intra-abdominal pathology.

D) Electrodiagnostic studies should be considered on at least 2 limbs. The testing should be performed by a medically trained physician (Neurologist or Physical Medicine & Rehabilitation specialist) with certification by the American Board of Electrodiagnostic Medicine.

II. **For the patient with IDENTIFIED RISK FACTORS (Table 2). Focus on nature of identified risk factors.**

A) Obesity or past history of obesity with bypass surgery or major abdominal surgery: Focus on nutritional deficiencies such as vitamin, trace minerals, diabetes, and endocrine abnormalities.Multi-limb electrodiagnostics is recommended.

B) Systemic illnesses: ESR, CRP, specific inflammatory markers for RA, Lupus, etc. Look for end-organ damage as painful peripheral neuropathies more common with disease advancement. Multi-limb electrodiagnostics is advised.

C) Infectious: HIV, hepatitis screen, test for immune competence. Check history for tropical/foreign exposures and test accordingly.

D) Inflammatory Bowel disease: Look for nutritional deficiencies, trace minerals, and inflammatory markers.

E) When etiology is unclear or concern is present for psychiatric issues, it is recommended that a thorough battery of psychometric testing be performed (MMPI-II, Millon clinical multiaxial inventory etc.) by a trained mental health professional to evaluate for evidence of factitious disorder, malingering, somatoform disorder, personality disorders, etc. The impact of emotional disturbances on physical complaints is well recognized and should not be dismissed as a portion of the clinical evaluation.

F) Toxic Etiology: including alcohol, solvents, insecticides, and metals. Perform appropriate lab studies to document exposure and end organ damage.

G) Pharmacologic Etiology: If suspected, obtain a list of all medication, including prescription, over-the-counter, nutritional and herbal supplements, medical foods, dietary patterns, alcohol, illicit substances, tobacco, etc. and evaluate for drug-drug interactions. Co-morbid states may mask interactions, as patients may be treating with multiple providers and overlapping prescriptions. Enlisting help of family members may be warranted.

H) Neoplastic Etiology: Cancer and paraneoplastic syndromes may be productive of an array of complaints including PPN. Suspicion and thorough evaluation is favored.

Table 4b:

III. When the initial evaluation is INCONCLUSIVE OR NEGATIVE

A strong suspicion of SFN should be considered, as this condition is often idiopathic, and symptoms can be vague. Consider EMG/NCS of multiple limbs, quantitative sensory testing, quantitative sudomotor axon reflex test (QSART), and skin biopsy looking for decreased alpha-delta and C fiber content, indicative of the SFN.

A 2 hour GTT and fasting blood sugar along with lipid panel should be performed based on a strong association between SFN, hyperlipidemia and abnormal GTT. The physical exam is almost always normal, except for complaints of unverifiable sensory abnormalities.

Quantitative Sensory Testing (QST) may be obtained, but the results are based on subjective responses and are not always helpful. QSART measures postganglionic sympathetic cholinergic function. A 73% sensitivity in SFN has been reported and may reflect early sudomotor dysfunction.[79]

Skin biopsy can provide objective evaluation of small nerve fiber concentration. This is performed as a punch biopsy, often of the area of greatest involvement. The biopsy provides quantification of small fiber (alpha-delta and C fibers) at the dermal-epidermal junction. This test has a reported sensitivity of 78-92% and a specificity of 65-90%. This biopsy may assess accurately the presence of SFN, but not its' etiology.[79]

Performing multiple diagnostics in tandem may provide an overall more accurate assessment of SFN presence.

Symptoms should be addressed cautiously. Diminish narcotic use due to complications, and keep polypharmacy at a minimum to avoid potential drug-drug interactions. If symptoms remain over 6-8 weeks, another history and exam should be performed and compared to original to assess objective changes and/or progression.

The possibility of a psychiatric diagnosis (e.g. somatoform disorder, factitious disorder, depressive disorder, anxiety disorder, personality disorder, malingering) causing or contributing to symptoms should be considered when physical explanation is elusive. This concept is best addressed by consulting a mental health profession, skilled in the performance and interpretation of psychometric tests.

Finally, consultation with appropriate medical specialists including Rheumatology, Neurology, Endocrinology, or General Internal Medicine is always a good consideration when assessing causes of systemic symptoms.

Section 5 (Physical) References

1.   Marinus J, Moseley GL, Birklein F, et al. Clinical features and pathophysiology of complex regional pain syndrome. Lancet Neurol. 2011;10(7):637-648.

2.   Chowdhury D, Patel N. Approach to a case of autonomic peripheral neuropathy. J Assoc Physicians India. 2006;54:727-732.

3.   McDougall AJ, McLeod JG. Autonomic neuropathy, II: Specific peripheral neuropathies. J Neurol Sci. 1996;138(1-2):1-13.

4.   Freeman R. Autonomic peripheral neuropathy. Lancet. 2005;365(9466):1259-1270.

5.   Grantz M, Huan MC. Unusual peripheral neuropathies. part I: Extrinsic causes. Semin Neurol. 2010;30(4):387-395.

6.   Azhary H, Farooq MU, Bhanushali M, Majid A, Kassab MY. Peripheral neuropathy: Differential diagnosis and management. Am Fam Physician. 2010;81(7):887-892.

7.   Grantz M. Unusual peripheral neuropathies. part III: Intrinsic inherited causes. Semin Neurol. 2010;30(4):405-415.

8.   Chaudhry V, Cornblath DR, Corse A, Freimer M, Simmons-O'Brien E, Vogelsang G. Thalidomide-induced neuropathy. Neurology. 2002;59(12):1872-1875.

9.   Manji H. Drug-induced neuropathies. Handb Clin Neurol. 2013;115:729-742.

10.   Kucera P, Balaz M, Varsik P, Kurca E. Pathogenesis of alcoholic neuropathy. Bratisl Lek Listy. 2002;103(1):26-29.

11. Dina OA, Khasar SG, Alessandri-Haber N, Green PG, Messing RO, Levine JD. Alcohol-induced stress in painful alcoholic neuropathy. Eur J Neurosci. 2008;27(1):83-92.

12. Chaudhry V, Umapathi T, Ravich WJ. Neuromuscular diseases and disorders of the alimentary system. Muscle Nerve. 2002;25(6):768-784.

13. Koike H, Sobue G. Alcoholic neuropathy. Curr Opin Neurol. 2006;19(5):481-486.

14. Thomson RM, Parry GJ. Neuropathies associated with excessive exposure to lead. Muscle Nerve. 2006;33(6):732-741.

15. Marrs TC. Organophosphate poisoning. Pharmacol Ther. 1993;58(1):51-66.

16. Balali-Mood M, Balali-Mood K. Neurotoxic disorders of organophosphorus compounds and their managements. Arch Iran Med. 2008;11(1):65-89.

17. Dick FD. Solvent neurotoxicity. Occup Environ Med. 2006;63(3):221-6, 179.

18. Pace A, Giannarelli D, Galie E, et al. Vitamin E neuroprotection for cisplatin neuropathy: A randomized, placebo-controlled trial. Neurology. 2010;74(9):762-766.

19. Chaudhry V, Chaudhry M, Crawford TO, Simmons-O'Brien E, Griffin JW. Toxic neuropathy in patients with pre-existing neuropathy. Neurology. 2003;60(2):337-340.

20. Manji H. Toxic neuropathy. Curr Opin Neurol. 2011;24(5):484-490.

21.   Mateos MV, Bringhen S, Richardson PG, et al. Bortezomib cumulative dose, efficacy, and tolerability with three different bortezomib-melphalan-prednisone regimens in previously untreated myeloma patients ineligible for high-dose therapy. Haematologica. 2014;99(6):1114-1122.

22.   Rather ZA, Chowta MN, Prakash Raju GJ, Mubeen F. Evaluation of the adverse reactions of antiretroviral drug regimens in a tertiary care hospital. Indian J Pharmacol. 2013;45(2):145-148.

23.   Tierney EF, Thurman DJ, Beckles GL, Cadwell BL. Association of statin use with peripheral neuropathy in the U.S. population 40 years of age or older. J Diabetes. 2013;5(2):207-215.

24.   Baima J, Krivickas L. Evaluation and treatment of peroneal neuropathy. Curr Rev Musculoskelet Med. 2008;1(2):147-153.

25.   Baumgaertel MW, Kraemer M, Berlit P. Neurologic complications of acute and chronic renal disease. Handb Clin Neurol. 2014;119:383-393.

26.   Bansal VK, Bansal S. Nervous system disorders in dialysis patients. Handb Clin Neurol. 2014;119:395-404.

27.   Kelkar P. Diabetic neuropathy. Semin Neurol. 2005;25(2):168-173.

28.   Mattie R, Irwin RW. Neurosarcoidosis presenting as mononeuritis multiplex. Am J Phys Med Rehabil. 2014;93(4):349-354.

29.   Kawakami T, Okudaira A, Okano T, et al. Treatment for cutaneous arteritis patients with mononeuritis multiplex and elevated C-reactive protein. J Dermatol. 2013;40(12):955-961.

30.   Bove D, Lupoli A, Caccavale S, Piccolo V, Ruocco E. Dermatological and immunological conditions due to nerve lesions. Funct Neurol. 2013;28(2):83-91.

31.   Streifler JY, Molad Y. Connective tissue disorders: Systemic lupus erythematosus, sjogren's syndrome, and scleroderma. Handb Clin Neurol. 2014;119:463-473.

32.   Al-Homood IA. Rheumatic conditions in patients with diabetes mellitus. Clin Rheumatol. 2013;32(5):527-533.

33.   Grantz M. Unusual peripheral neuropathies. part II: Intrinsic reactive causes. Semin Neurol. 2010;30(4):396-404.

34.   Oomatia A, Fang H, Petri M, Birnbaum J. Peripheral neuropathies in systemic lupus erythematosus: Clinical features, disease associations, and immunologic characteristics evaluated over a twenty-five-year study period. Arthritis Rheumatol. 2014;66(4):1000-1009.

35.   Ostrowski RA, Takagishi T, Robinson J. Rheumatoid arthritis, spondyloarthropathies, and relapsing polychondritis. Handb Clin Neurol. 2014;119:449-461.

36.   Vrancken AF, Said G. Vasculitic neuropathy. Handb Clin Neurol. 2013;115:463-483.

37.   Ashok Muley S, Brown K, Parry GJ. Paraneoplastic vasculitic neuropathy related to carcinoid tumor. J Neurol. 2008;255(7):1085-1087.

38.   Moris G. Inflammatory bowel disease: An increased risk factor for neurologic complications. World J Gastroenterol. 2014;20(5):1228-1237.

39.   Singh S, Kumar N, Loftus EV,Jr, Kane SV. Neurologic complications in patients with inflammatory bowel disease: Increasing relevance in the era of biologics. Inflamm Bowel Dis. 2013;19(4):864-872.

40.   Evans NE, Turner MR. Neurogastroentrology: An A to Z. Pract Neurol. 2011;11(4):220-230.

41.	Bouskela E, Kraemer de Aguiar LG, Nivoit P, Bahia LR, Villela NR, Bottino DA. Vascular dysfunction in metabolic disorders: Evaluation of some therapeutic interventions. Bull Acad Natl Med. 2007;191(3):475-92; discussion 492-3.

42.	Simpson DM. Selected peripheral neuropathies associated with human immunodeficiency virus infection and antiretroviral therapy. J Neurovirol. 2002;8 Suppl 2:33-41.

43.	Verma R, Lalla R, Babu S. Mononeuritis multiplex and painful ulcers as the initial manifestation of hepatitis B infection. BMJ Case Rep. 2013;2013:10.1136/bcr-2013-009666.

44.	Yuki N, Yoshioka A, Yasuda R, Ohmichi T, Oka N. Hepatitis C virus-associated neuropathy accompanied by eosinophilic vasculitis and gran uloma formation. Intern Med. 2014;53(11):1187-1190.

45.	Cacoub P, Terrier B, Saadoun D. Hepatitis C virus-induced vasculitis: Therapeutic options. Ann Rheum Dis. 2014;73(1):24-30.

46.	Sellner J, Steiner I. Neurologic complications of hepatic viruses. Handb Clin Neurol. 2014;123:647-661.

47.	Gabbai AA, Castelo A, Oliveira AS. HIV peripheral neuropathy. Handb Clin Neurol. 2013;115:515-529.

48.	Krumina A, Logina I, Donaghy M, et al. Diphtheria with polyneuropathy in a closed community despite receiving recent booster vaccination. J Neurol Neurosurg Psychiatry. 2005;76(11):1555-1557.

49.	Sanghi V. Neurologic manifestations of diphtheria and pertussis. Handb Clin Neurol. 2014;121:1355-1359.

50.   Roman GC. Tropical myelopathies. Handb Clin Neurol. 2014;121:1521-1548.

51.   Serban AL, Udrea GF. Rheumatic manifestations in diabetic patients. J Med Life. 2012;5(3):252-257.

52.   Kelkar P, Parry GJ. Mononeuritis multiplex in diabetes mellitus: Evidence for underlying immune pathogenesis. J Neurol Neurosurg Psychiatry. 2003;74(6):803-806.

53.   Smith AG, Singleton JR. Impaired glucose tolerance and neuropathy. Neurologist. 2008;14(1):23-29.

54.   Muley SA, Parry GJ, Ercan-Fang NG. Isolated bibrachial plexopathy in a patient with type 2 diabetes. Diabetes Care. 2005;28(10):2591-2592.

55.   Vinik AI, Erbas T. Diabetic autonomic neuropathy. Handb Clin Neurol. 2013;117:279-294.

56.   Godil A, Berriman D, Knapik S, Norman M, Godil F, Firek AF. Diabetic neuropathic cachexia. West J Med. 1996;165(6):382-385.

57.   Said G, Lacroix C, Lozeron P, Ropert A, Plante V, Adams D. Inflammatory vasculopathy in multifocal diabetic neuropathy. Brain. 2003;126(Pt 2):376-385.

58.   Said G. Diabetic neuropathy--a review. Nat Clin Pract Neurol. 2007;3(6):331-340.

59.   McDougall AJ, McLeod JG. Autonomic neuropathy, I. clinical features, investigation, pathophysiology, and treatment. J Neurol Sci. 1996;137(2):79-88.

60.   England JD, Gronseth GS, Franklin G, et al. Evaluation of distal symmetric polyneuropathy: The role of laboratory and genetic testing (an evidence-based review). Muscle Nerve. 2009;39(1):116-125.

61.   Gallagher G, Rabquer A, Kerber K, Calabek B, Callaghan B. Value of thyroid and rheumatologic studies in the evaluation of peripheral neuropathy. Neurol Clin Pract. 2013;3(2):90-98.

62.   Frantz DJ. Neurologic complications of bariatric surgery: Involvement of central, peripheral, and enteric nervous systems. Curr Gastroenterol Rep. 2012;14(4):367-372.

63.   Folope V, Coeffier M, Dechelotte P. Nutritional deficiencies associated with bariatric surgery. Gastroenterol Clin Biol. 2007;31(4):369-377.

64.   Kaidar-Person O, Rosenthal RJ. Malnutrition in morbidly obese patients: Fact or fiction? Minerva Chir. 2009;64(3):297-302.

65.   Callaghan B, Feldman E. The metabolic syndrome and neuropathy: Therapeutic challenges and opportunities. Ann Neurol. 2013;74(3):397-403.

66.   Toh SY, Zarshenas N, Jorgensen J. Prevalence of nutrient deficiencies in bariatric patients. Nutrition. 2009;25(11-12):1150-1156.

67.   Schweiger C, Weiss R, Berry E, Keidar A. Nutritional deficiencies in bariatric surgery candidates. Obes Surg. 2010;20(2):193-197.

68.   Ba F, Siddiqi ZA. Neurologic complications of bariatric surgery. Rev Neurol Dis. 2010;7(4):119-124.

69.   Becker DA, Balcer LJ, Galetta SL. The neurological complications of nutritional deficiency following bariatric surgery. J Obes. 2012;2012:608534.

70.   Koch TR, Finelli FC. Postoperative metabolic and nutritional complications of bariatric surgery. Gastroenterol Clin North Am. 2010;39(1):109-124.

71.   Sachedina S, Toth C. Progression in idiopathic, diabetic, paraproteinemic, alcoholic, and B12 deficiency neuropathy. J Peripher Nerv Syst. 2013;18(3):247-255.

72.   Alvarez-Leite JI. Nutrient deficiencies secondary to bariatric surgery. Curr Opin Clin Nutr Metab Care. 2004;7(5):569-575.

73.   Berger JR, Singhal D. The neurologic complications of bariatric surgery. Handb Clin Neurol. 2014;120:587-594.

74.   Pfeiffer RF. Neurologic manifestations of malabsorption syndromes. Handb Clin Neurol. 2014;120:621-632.

75.   Kazemi A, Frazier T, Cave M. Micronutrient-related neurologic complications following bariatric surgery. Curr Gastroenterol Rep. 2010;12(4):288-295.

76.   Hoitsma E, Reulen JP, de Baets M, Drent M, Spaans F, Faber CG. Small fiber neuropathy: A common and important clinical disorder. J Neurol Sci. 2004;227(1):119-130.

77.   Zhou L, Li J, Ontaneda D, Sperling J. Metabolic syndrome in small fiber sensory neuropathy. J Clin Neuromuscul Dis. 2011;12(4):235-243.

78.   Eslamian F, Bahrami A, Aghamohammadzadeh N, Niafar M, Salekzamani Y, Behkamrad K. Electrophysiologic changes in patients with untreated primary hypothyroidism. J Clin Neurophysiol. 2011;28(3):323-328.

79.   Hovaguimian A, Gibbons CH. Diagnosis and treatment of pain in small fiber neuropathy. Curr Pain Headache Rep 2011 June; 15(3): 193-200.

80.   Tesfaye S, et al. Vascular risk factors and diabetes. NEJM. 2005; 352;4: 341-350.

Non-Physical

Scientific findings indicate that it is usually misdirected to separate consideration of different types of chronic benign pain presentations from one another, or to separate consideration of chronic pain complaints for different parts of the body from one another (misdirected in terms of both science and health care)[8,9].

In terms of scientific credibility, and in terms of maximizing the chance of health care being beneficial for the pain complaints, it is better to consider any and all pain complaints and other physical complaints, which do not have a clear general medical cause, as portions of a clinical presentation which has a unifying theme involving the individual's personality.

Consequently, risk factors for almost any type of chronic benign pain complaints will be of relevance to the differential diagnostic process for a claim of complex regional pain syndrome. The significance of the relevance to the differential diagnostic process in CRPS claims cannot be underscored with more emphasis.[5-9]

Certain fundamental considerations should be kept in mind when the differential diagnostic process is undertaken by any clinician. As a result of several comprehensive reviews of claim behavior by patients who present with this possible construct, any clinician who is faced with a claim of complex regional pain syndrome would be wise and justified to reject that diagnostic claim, even in the absence of a comprehensive differential diagnostic workup.

Previous publications have made several discreet points when analyzing the claim process in the individual who is presenting with a possible CRPS diagnosis.[6,7]

The construct of complex regional pain syndrome has not been validated as corresponding to any actual health condition. It probably cannot be validated, given the abnormal way in which the construct was created, and the unreliability of the construct[6,7,11,12]. A diagnosis which involves any of the differentials will probably have more credibility than a diagnosis of complex regional pain syndrome.

Clinical presentations of relevance to the complex regional pain syndrome construct are reportedly extremely rare. Consequently, any of the differentials is far more probable for any individual case (far more probable than complex regional pain syndrome is said to be). Examples have been published that describe the manner in which differentials are much more probable than complex regional pain syndrome is said to be.[6,7]

All of the objectively verifiable issues that have been written into the construct of complex regional pain syndrome can be created through disuse[6,7]. Disuse has been specified as the apparent link between psychological and social issues, and clinical presentations which involve such objectively verifiable issues. One example is that psychopathology and/or social influences lead to abnormal patterns of disuse, and that disuse then leads to the objectively verifiable abnormalities.[15,23] Therefore, the list of differentials that is included at the end of this section is not comprehensive. Any other issue which might prompt disuse should also be considered.

Patients are not reliable reporters of their own histories. The unreliability is especially pronounced when the patient seeks or obtains financial compensation for their complaints.[3,5] Scientific findings have repeatedly indicated that the vast majority of people who obtain a complex regional pain syndrome diagnosis will be in a compensation context.[1,24,25] Consequently, historical reports from such individuals cannot be credibly considered to be reliable or accurate. Therefore, a differential diagnostic process which is only based on information gained directly from the patient/examinee will not be credible. The process should instead involve an effort to obtain and review a comprehensive set of records from the individual's entire life including the following: health care, education, military, occupational, legal, etc. Such a review of records will probably be the most important part of the process. The process should also include utilization of a credible diagnostic methodology for every differential issue on the list at the end of this section plus every differential issue that has been previously identified within this paper.

Historically, diagnostic methodology called for complex regional pain syndrome to be excluded from diagnostic consideration if any other potential explanation for the clinical presentation could be identified. Similarly, such standards indicated that a diagnosis of complex regional pain syndrome would not be credible unless every other potential explanation for the clinical presentation had been credibly ruled out. While this historical aspect of the construct has been violated by some modern conceptualizations (see Appendix A), it is still recommended that the historical approach be maintained in any individual case.

SUMMARY LIST OF COMMONLY RELEVANT
DIFFERENTIAL DIAGNOSTIC CONSIDERATIONS

- Eligibility for financial compensation (or efforts to obtain financial compensation)

    o Scientific findings have indicated that this is the dominant risk factor for chronic pain claims in general. Scientific findings have additionally indicated that complex regional pain syndrome claims are an especially good example of the strong association between such compensation issues and chronic pain.[6-9,24]

- Psychopathology that would have traditionally fallen into the category of somatoform disorders, and/or a history of other pain complaints and physical complaints

    o As of 2013, the American Psychiatric Association's primary textbook[20] specified that this category of mental illness had been especially well-validated scientifically, and has been recognized as having been extensively validated for decades. In spite of that published report from the American Psychiatric Association, the same Association discontinued this category of mental illness in 2013.[2] Consequently, diagnosticians are warned that the 2013 version of the American Psychiatric Association's diagnostic system does not provide a method for addressing this differential diagnostic issue. Note should be made that the American

Psychiatric Association's new construct entitled "Somatic Symptom and Related Disorders" is especially insufficient for applying the relevant scientific knowledge base to any individual case. The diagnostician will have to turn directly to the scientific knowledge base and to other diagnostic methods, in order to address this differential diagnostic issue. Such efforts are warranted due to scientific findings that individuals who receive a complex regional pain syndrome diagnosis are even more somatoform in their presentation than are chronic pain patients who do not obtain such a diagnosis[13]

o Scientific findings have indicated that previous pain complaints, pain complaints that are not part of the complex regional pain syndrome claim (even if they do not precede the issues that are part of the complex regional pain syndrome claim), and other physical complaints (e.g. palpitations/extra heartbeats, breathing difficulties, diarrhea, constipation, eczema, tiredness, dizziness, etc.) are predictive of the development of new chronic pain complaints[8,9]. Of special relevance to the current discussion, the example can be offered of migraine headaches being specifically predictive of an individual obtaining a diagnosis of complex regional pain syndrome. Such scientific findings overlap with scientific findings regarding forms of psychopathology which historically were categorized as somatoform disorders. Consequently, the diagnostician can often adequately address this portion of the differential diagnostic process based on a review of such previous complaints and other complaints (without fully applying the scientific knowledge base regarding psychopathology which was historically categorized as somatoform).

• Factitious disorder or malingering

o Publications have emerged which indicate that many patients who obtain a diagnosis of complex regional pain syndrome demonstrate an invalid clinical presentation when objectively assessed.[6,7,19] It is further postulated that such patients even deliberately create such presentations.[21] Given the repeated scientific findings indicating that the vast majority of such patients will be in a compensation context, such patients will usually not be eligible for a factitious disorder diagnosis. Diagnostic standards instead call for the adoption of a strong suspicion of malingering when a factitious-like patient is in a compensation context.[2] Any consistencies between an individual presentation and factitious disorder should receive intense consideration, at least because of the high rate of death that has been established for factitious-like individuals who file compensation claims.[17]

- Personality disorders

- Psychopathology that would have traditionally fallen into the category of anxiety disorders

  o The category of anxiety disorders was drastically changed in the 2013 version of the American Psychiatric Association's diagnostic system.[2] Similarly, relevant diagnostic concepts and protocols were drastically altered.[2] Consequently, the diagnostician might need to consider diagnostic protocols from modern categories. The new categories include those entitled "Anxiety Disorders", "Obsessive-Compulsive and Related Disorders", and "Trauma- and Stressor-Related Disorders." There should also be consideration given to protocols from other diagnostic systems or the original research protocols from studies which revealed the strong relationship of such psychopathology to complex regional pain syndrome-like presentations, and to chronic pain complaints in general. Such extensive effort is necessary, given scientific findings which indicated that a vulnerability to anxiety is one of the best predictors of the development of a complex regional pain syndrome-like presentation.

- Psychopathology that would have traditionally fallen into the category of mood disorders

  - The category of mood disorders was eliminated by the introduction of the 2013 version of the American Psychiatric Association's diagnostic system and relevant diagnostic concepts and protocols were drastically altered.[2] Consequently, the diagnostician might need to consider diagnostic protocols from multiple modern categories including the new categories entitled "Depressive Disorders" and "Bipolar and Related Disorder." There should also be consideration given to protocols from other diagnostic systems, and the original research protocols from studies which revealed the strong relationship of such psychopathology to complex regional pain syndrome-like presentations, and to chronic pain complaints in general. Such efforts are warranted given scientific findings which indicated that complex regional pain syndrome-like presentations are overwhelmingly associated with pre-existing psychopathology that would have historically fallen within the category of mood disorders.

- Psychopathology that would have traditionally fallen into the category of substance- related disorders

  - The category of substance-related disorders was re-titled and conceptually altered to a drastic extent by the introduction of the 2013 version of the American Psychiatric Association's diagnostic system. While previous editions of that system deliberately avoided utilization of any construct which could be labeled as "addiction", the new system embraces such a construct – and even embraces that construct for issues that do not involve substances. Similarly, relevant diagnostic concepts and protocols were drastically altered.[2] Consequently, the diagnostician might need to consider protocols from the new category of "Substance-Related and Addictive Disorders," other diagnostic systems, and the original research protocols from studies which revealed the strong relationship of such psychopathology to chronic pain complaints.

- Psychotic disorders

  - o The category for psychotic disorders was re-titled and substantially altered by the introduction of the 2013 version of the American Psychiatric Association's diagnostic system. Additionally, diagnostic concepts and protocols were substantially altered.[2] Consequently, the diagnostician might need to consider protocols from the new category of "Schizophrenia Spectrum and Other Psychotic Disorders", other diagnostic systems, and the original research protocols from studies which revealed the strong relationship of such psychopathology to chronic pain complaints.

- A history of narcotic medication/opiate/opioid consumption

  - o Readers should note that the effects of narcotic medication/opiate/opioid consumption parallel many of the otherwise unexplainable issues that have been written into the construct of complex regional pain syndrome.[4]

- Chronic pain as a learned phenomenon (central sensitization), which can be unlearned.

  - o The realization that chronic pain can actually be a learned phenomenon has now been extensively reviewed. Evaluation and treatment of these patients requires a substantial effort in multifactorial identification of sensitization issues and motivation.[8,9,18]

- o Relevant scientific findings highlight the need for differential diagnostic efforts to go beyond the individual patient, by including consideration of any family history of pain complaints, chronic health problems, disability claims, and any other sources from which such issues could have been learned.

- Smoking

- Obesity

- Childhood abuse and neglect

- Excessive and/or misdirected healthcare (e.g., healthcare efforts that have been focused on attempting to directly alleviate chronic pain)

- Being away from work

Section 5 (non-physical) References:

1. Allen G, Galer BS, Schwartz L. Epidemiology of complex regional pain syndrome: a retrospective chart review of 134 patients. Pain. 1999; 80 (3); 539-544.

2. American Psychiatric Association: *Diagnostic and Statistical Manual of Mental Disorders. Fifth Edition.* Washington, DC: American Psychiatric Association, 2013.

3. Barth RJ. Claimant-Reported History is Not a Credible Basis for Clinical or Administrative Decision-Making. *The Guides Newsletter*, September/October, 2009. American Medical Association.

4. Barth RJ. Prescription narcotics: An obstacle to maximum medical improvement. *The Guides Newsletter*, March/April, 2011a. American Medical Association.

5. Barth RJ. Claimant-Reported History is Not a Credible Basis for Clinical or Administrative Decision-Making. In: Melhorn JM and Talmage JB. *13th Annual American Academy of Orthopaedic Surgeons Occupational Orthopaedics and Workers Compensation: A Multidisciplinary Perspective.* 2011b. American Academy of Orthopaedic Surgeons.

6. Barth RJ and Haralson R. Differential Diagnosis for Complex Regional Pain Syndrome.*The Guides Newsletter,* September/October 2007a. American Medical Association.

7. Barth RJ and Haralson R. Differential Diagnosis for Complex Regional Pain Syndrome.in: Melhorn JM and Shields NN. *9th Annual Occupational Orthopaedics and Workers Compensation: A Multidisciplinary Perspective.* 2007b. American Academy of Orthopaedic Surgeons.

8. Barth RJ. Chronic Pain: Fundamental Scientific Considerations, Specifically for Legal Claims. *AMA Guides Newsletter*, Jan/Feb 2013a. American Medical Association.

9. Barth RJ. Chronic Pain: Fundamental Scientific Considerations, Specifically For Legal Claims. Chapter M in: Melhorn JM (editor). *16th Annual American Academy of Orthopaedic Surgeons Occupational Orthopaedics and Workers Compensation: A Multidisciplinary Perspective*. 2014. American Academy of Orthopaedic Surgeons.

10. Bass C. Complex regional pain syndrome medicalises limb pain. British Medical Journal. 2014 Apr 28;348:g2631.

11. Biller, J (Chair), et al. Neuropathic pain and Iatrogenesis. Pages 91-104 in: Iatrogenic Neurology, Continuum, 7, 2, 2001. American Academy of Neurology.

12. Borchers AT, Gershwin ME. Complex regional pain syndrome: a comprehensive and critical review. Autoimmun Rev. 2014 Mar;13(3):242-65.

13. Bruehl S, Husfeldt B, Lubenow TR, Nath H, Ivankovich AD. Psychological differences between reflex sympathetic dystrophy and non-RSD chronic pain patients. *Pain*. 1996 Sep;67(1):107-14.

14. Butler SH: Disuse and CRPS, in Harden RN, Baron R, Janig W (Eds): *Complex Regional Pain Syndrome*. Seattle, WA: IASP Press, 2001, pp 141-150.

15. Cocchiarella, L. and Andersson, G. (editors) (2001). *Guides to the Evaluation of Permanent Impairment, Fifth Edition*. American Medical Association.

16. Del Piñal F. Editorial. I have a dream ... reflex sympathetic dystrophy (RSD or Complex Regional Pain Syndrome - CRPS I) does not exist. J Hand Surg Eur Vol. 2013 Jul;38(6):595-7.

17. Eisendrath SJ & McNiel DE. Factitious Physical Disorders, Litigation, and Mortality. Psychosomatics: Journal of Consultation Liaison Psychiatry. 45(4), Aug 2004, 350-353.

18. Flor H, & Turk DC. Chronic Pain/an Integrated Biobehavioral Approach. International Association for the Study of Pain. 2011.

19. Greiffenstein M, Gervais R, Baker WJ, Artiola L, Smith H. Symptom validity testing in medically unexplained pain: a chronic regional pain syndrome type 1 case series. The Clinical Psychologist. 2013;27(1):138-47.

20. Hales RE, Yudofsky SC, Gabbard GO (editors). The American Psychiatric Publishing Textbook of Psychiatry, Fifth Edition. American Psychiatric Publishing, Inc., 2008.

21. Mailis-Gagnon A, Nicholson K, Blumberger D, Zurowski M. Characteristics and period prevalence of self-induced disorder in patients referred to a pain clinic with the diagnosis of complex regional pain syndrome. *Clin J Pain*. 2008 Feb;24(2):176-85.

22. Ring D, Barth R, and Barsky A. Evidence-based medicine: disproportionate pain and disability, *Journal of Hand Surgery*, volume 34a, August 2010, 1345-1347.

23. Rondinelli RD, Brigham CR, Genovese E, et al. (Editors). *Guides to the Evaluation of Permanent Impairment Sixth Edition (Second Printing)*. American Medical Association, 2009.

24. Talmage JB, Melhorn JM, Ackerman WE, & Barth RJ. Musculoskeletal Disorders: Conditions of Uncertain Pathophysiology – Acute and Chronic Pain, in: Melhorn, JM, et al. (editors). *Guides to the Evaluation of Disease and Injury Causation, Second Edition*. 2013. American Medical Association.

25. Verdugo RJ and Ochoa JL. Abnormal movements in complex regional pain syndrome: assessment of their nature. Muscle & Nerve. 2000; 23 (2), 198-205.

Section 6

A Critical Review of Treatments

Establishing evidence based treatment guidelines for CRPS has, at least to this point, been an exercise akin to the search for the Fountain of Youth. Two major evidence based practice guidelines that are widely used in the management of workers compensation patients have gone on record indicating that there is no current literature support for any treatments for CRPS[1-2]. Of course, the practitioner is not served by having a blank chapter when dealing with evidence based answers, but it is an important point to make.

The American College of Occupational and Environmental Medicine (ACOEM) Practice Guidelines postulates that the reason that there is no EBM answers to CRPS treatment lies primarily in that research done on the subject does not use diagnostic criteria uniformly, and that population of patients who have been labeled as having CRPS are often not uniform. This lack of adherence to consistency will automatically lead to questions regarding the quality of any study looking at CRPS treatments. Additionally, ACOEM states that because of what they describe as "advocagenic issues," it is nearly impossible to even consider randomized controlled studies for these patients due to the overwhelming involvement with disability systems and liability claims that accompany the diagnosis.

The Official Disability Guidelines Treatment in Workers Compensation (ODG) evidence based guidelines, as well as ACOEM, makes another critical point when discussing CRPS treatment literature in that so many studies look at pain control or pain relief as opposed to functional improvement. In many studies, a "successful" treatment is patient-defined by a reduction of pain by 50% without any eye turned toward functional improvement. Obviously, when evaluating treatment success and failure it is best to rely upon the objective rather than the subjective.

As various groups such as ODG, ACOEM, and others have wrestled with these issues, trends over the last 5 years would indicate that there is a turn more toward functional restoration as opposed to pain treatment modalities in patients who have been given the CRPS diagnosis[3]. Of all treatment options available, consensus amongst these various guidelines seem to fall within hierarchy of three general areas (listed in order of importance): rehabilitation, psychological treatment, and pain management.

Rehabilitation

The general trend of recommendations in this area can be summed up in what is frequently described as a "use it or lose it" perspective. Most studies continually refer to the fact that education of the patient is paramount in this respect and that better long term outcomes occur when the patient is encouraged to use the extremity with CRPS as "normally" as possible, including use for work tasks[4]. There is some debate regarding the best methodology to employ in order to get the CRPS patient to use the extremity, but graded exercise programs and mirror therapy seems to be slightly better than other rehabilitation options including that of strengthening, desensitization techniques, yoga, recreational activities and unique approaches such as scrub brush exercises[5-6].

It is frequently pointed out that a creation of a "therapeutic alliance" is necessary regarding rehabilitation professionals who treat CRPS patients. A rehabilitation professional (OT or PT) with some experience and expertise in these areas is often helpful because some of the therapeutic activities might temporarily increase pain (at least initially) and the presentation of the diagnosis is often within the scope of a liability or disability benefit system[2].

Psychological Treatment

With such a high incidence of psychiatric co-morbidity seen with CRPS patients, the patient labeled with CRPS should be evaluated psychologically early on to investigate for other potential factors that maintain chronic pain behavior and disability[7-9].

Most consensus guidelines indicate that cognitive behavioral therapy is helpful for CRPS patients. This therapy should be focused on improved quality of life, development of pain coping skills, improving facilitation of other modalities and vocational counseling.[10] If an Axis I diagnosis is determined, then it should be definitively addressed and treated (anxiety disorder, major depressive disorder, bipolar disorder, post-traumatic stress disorder).

Pain Management

Absent in many guidelines and published papers is the importance of the two strategies listed above regarding "pain management". Most guidelines and literature reviews look at the subject of "pain management" only from the perspective of medications, injections or surgical procedures, when an interdisciplinary approach is required.

When talking about oral medications, it is important to note that the role of medication should be to increase the goals of rehabilitation as stated above including the natural outcome being a return to function. Any treatment strategy that is focused upon pain alone is doomed to fail.

With those thoughts in mind, we must also be cognizant that the literature regarding medications and interventional procedures is often extrapolated from studies dealing with neurological pain disorders and chronic musculoskeletal disorders (such as low back pain). There are simply very few scattered studies that directly speak to CRPS. Most medications have limited effectiveness.

It is helpful to think about medications from the perspective of what it is that one is actually treating. To that end, the recommendations regarding medication effectiveness generally follow these parameters:

1. Regional inflammatory reaction: Non-steroidal anti-inflammatory drugs (NSAIDS) seem to have some benefit, but it is questionable as to dosing, intervals and duration of use. It is possible that they have benefit not because of their inflammatory control properties but because of pain pathway properties. Oral corticosteroids are effective but only for short term use and early on in the treatment course. There is some evidence that topical DMSO, by its property as a free radical scavenger may have some utility especially when used as part of an active exercise program[11-13].

2. Stimulus-independent pain: Acetaminophen is generally considered a reasonable medication for use in treating CRPS. Although there is a paucity of literature on the subject, the general consensus is that as a relatively safe medication that is universally used for a variety of pain conditions, its helpfulness can be extrapolated here. The use of tricyclic

antidepressants, because of the excellent literature suggesting its improvement for patients with neuropathic pain, is generally accepted as an option for treating CRPS. However, less consensus exists regarding other anti-depressants such as SSRIs, SNRIs, or atypicals. Some guidelines suggest that these medication are helpful and others not[1, 14].

Anticonvulsants seem to be the one drug class where at least some reasonable studies exist that show improvement within CRPS patients. There seems to be slightly more support for gabapentin than any other drugs within this class[15-16].

A great deal of time and effort is spent on the topic of opioid use within most treatment guidelines, with an overwhelming discourse describing the negative consequences that can ensue with these medications. There is no evidence that these medications should be used routinely for CRPS. Most guidance continues to suggest that these medications can be helpful but ONLY if there is a regimented focus on appropriate patient selection, ONLY if functional improvement can be shown while on these medications and then ONLY if they are used for a short course[17-19].

3. Treatment of bone reabsorption and resultant pain: Perhaps the one exception to the rule regarding quality literature and CRPS treatments is in regard to bisphosphonate-type compounds and calcitonin. Bisphosphonates include alendronate, ibandronate, risedronate, zoledronate, etidronate, and pamidronate. There is no research on the newer longer-lasting drugs that are administered by periodic IV infusion (ibandronate, zoledronate, and pamidronate). Although the mechanism of action is uncertain as to how pain relief is created, significant improvement has been found in limited studies with intravenous alendronate. Alendronate (Fosamax®) given in oral doses of 40 mg a day (over an 8 week period) produced improvements in pain, pressure tolerance, and joint mobility. There has also been evidence of improvement of pain with pamidronate. It is important to note that osteopenia was not an outcome[20-21].

4. Injectable modifiers: Some injectable medications have been recommended for CRPS treatments. Regional blockade with clonidine, as an adjunct to other therapies seems to afford some benefit. There is some support for bretylium blocks, but only for severe   cases when basically nothing else has been helpful[22-23].

Yes, this is a relatively short list. A much longer list includes those preparations where the literature has shown no support for use in CRPS patients. Such medications include: herbal preparations, ketamine, ketanserin, amantadine, muscle relaxants, thalidomide, TNF-alpha blockers, botulinum toxin, baclofen, intrathecal injectables, lidocaine infusions, guanethedine blocks, phentolamine blocks, reserpine blocks, and dietary supplements. A host of other interventional strategies have found to be unhelpful including: hyperbaric oxygen, magnets, acupuncture, kinesiotaping, cryotherapy, diathermy, external radiation, infrared, ultrasound, laser therapy, osteopathic or chiropractic manipulation, manipulation under anesthesia, myofascial release, reflexology, Galvanic stimulation, H wave stimulation, Interferential therapy, ionotophoresis, electrical stimulation, PENS, and TENS[1-2].

Lastly, one cannot end this discussion without commenting upon the use of spinal cord stimulators (SCS). Given that sympathectomy has been a dismal failure for treating CRPS and is not recommended for consideration, other consensus derived guidelines have discussed the potential help that SCS might bring. Just as in the case of opioids, these documents generally spend an inordinate amount of time warning us regarding the importance of appropriate patient selection when considering SCS. All guidelines require psychological review (of course we suggest that on all CRPS patients). The trend in the literature seems to be that for a select few, short, or intermediate term, SCS can be helpful as an adjunct to more aggressive functional restoration rehabilitative efforts. There seems to be little support for SCS to be used as a long term strategy alone[24-25].

Section 6 References

1. Hegmann KT (editor) ACOEM's Occupational Medicine Practice Guidelines, 3rd Edition. Complex Regional Pain Syndrome. 827-828.

2. Novak S (chapter lead) Official Disability Guidelines Treatment in Workers Compensation. Pain. http://www.worklossdatainstitute.verioiponly.com/odgtwc/pain.htm Accessed 12/01/2014.

3. Perez RS et al. Evidence based guidelines for complex regional pain syndrome type 1. BMC Neurol. 2010; 10: 20.

4. Talmage JB Melhorn JM Hyman MH. AMA Guides to the Evaluation of Work Ability and Return to Work. American Medical Association. Chicago. 2011

5. Oerlemans HM et al. Pain and reduced mobility in complex regional pain syndrome I: outcome of a prospective randomized controlled clinical trial of adjuvant physical therapy versus occupational therapy. Pain. 1999; 80(9):1038-43.

6. De Jong VR Onghena P. Reduction of pain related fear in complex regional pain syndrome type I: the application of graded exercise in vivo. Pain. 2005;116(3):264-75

7. Gonzales VA Martelli MF Baker JM. Psychological assessment of persons with chronic pain. NeurReahbiliation. 2000;14(2):69-83.

8. Lebovits AH. The psychological assessment of patients with chronic pain. Curr Rev Pain. 2000:4(2):122-6.

9. Tuner JA Romano JM. Behavioral and Psychological Assessment of Chronic Pain Patients. New York: Raven Press; 1989.

10. Linton SJ et al. The effects of cognitive behavioral and physical therapy preventive interventions on pain-related sick leave: a randomized controlled trial. Clin J Pain. 2005:21(2):109-19.

11. Stanton-Hicks M. Complex Regional Pain Syndrome. In: Warfield CA, Bajwa JH. Principles and Practice of Pain Medicine. 2nd ed. McGraw-Hill; 2004.

12. Kalita J Vajpayee A Misra UK. Comparison of prednisolone with piroxicam in complex regional pain syndrome following stroke: a randomized controlled trail. QJM. 2006;99(2):89-95

13. Perez RS Zuurmond WW Bezemer PD et al. The treatment of complex regional pain syndrome type I with free radical scavengers: a randomized controlled study. Pain. 2003;102(3):297-307.

14. Pilowski I Hallett EC Bassett DL et al. A controlled study of amitriptyline in the treatment of chronic pain. Pain. 1982;14(2):169-179.

15. Wiffen P, Collins S, McQuay H, Carroll D, Jadad A, Moore A. Anticonvulsant drugs for acute and chronic pain. Cochrane Database Syst Rev. 2005 Jul 20;(3)

16. Serpell MG; Neuropathic pain study group. Gabapentin in neuropathic pain syndromes: a randomised, double-blind, placebo-controlled trial. Pain. 2002;99:557-66.

17. Eisenberg E, McNicol E, Carr DB. Opioids for neuropathic pain. Cochrane Database Syst Rev. 2006; 3

18. de Leon-Casasola O. New developments in the treatment algorithm for peripheral neuropathic pain. Pain Med. 2011;12 :S100-8.

19. Eisenberg E, McNicol ED, Carr DB. Efficacy and safety of opioid agonists in the treatment of neuropathic pain of nonmalignant origin: systematic review and meta-analysis of randomized controlled trials. JAMA. 2005 Jun 22;293(24):3043-52.

20. Manicourt DH, Brasseur JP, Boutsen Y, Depreseux G, Devogelaer JP. Role of alendronate in therapy for posttraumatic complex regional pain syndrome type I of the lower extremity. Arthritis Rheum. 2004 Nov;50(11):3690-7.

21. Robinson JN Sandom J Chapman PT. Efficacy of pamidronate in coplex regional pain syndrome type I. Pain Med. 2004;5(3):276-80.

22. Racuk RI Eisenach JC Jackson K et al. Epidural clonidine treatment for refractory reflex sympathetic dystrophy. Anesthesiology. 1993;79(6):1163-9.

23. Hord AH Rooks MD Stepehens BO et al. Intravenous regional bretylium and lidocaine for treatment of reflex sympathetic dystrophy: a randomized, double blinded, placebo controlled study. Reg Anesth Pain Med. 2004;29(5):408-412.

24. Mailis-Gagnon A, Furlan A, Sandoval J, Taylor R, Spinal cord stimulation for chronic pain, Cochrane Database Syst Rev. 2004;3:CD003783.

25. Taylor RS, Buyten JP, Buchser E. Spinal cord stimulation for complex regional pain syndrome: A systematic review of the clinical and cost-effectiveness literature and assessment of prognostic factors. Eur J Pain. 2006 Feb;10(2):91-101.

Section 7

The Medicolegal Context

Scientific findings have repeatedly demonstrated that, when a diagnosis of CRPS is made, the diagnosed individual has probably filed some kind of legal claim (e.g., personal injury claims, workers compensation claims) in regard to that diagnosis.[1,75,81] Scientific findings have indicated that such diagnoses are especially common in workers compensation claims.[75,81]

A possible reason for the especially strong association with workers compensation is that standards of evidence within many workers compensation systems are notoriously low. This allows a construct which has little, to no, scientific credibility (such as CRPS) to slip into workers compensation, even though it might not satisfy standards of evidence for other types of legal claims.

In regard to the manner in which cases that involve a diagnosis of complex regional pain syndrome are dominated by legal claims, the American Medical Association's AMA Guides to the Evaluation of Disease and Injury Causation notes: "An interesting and medically unexplainable concern is that occupational injury (Worker's Compensation) involves a minority of the total number of injuries that occur, and yet in published case series CRPS seems to be concentrated in compensation settings."[75] In one scientific sample, claims of workplace injury accounted for 80%of the diagnoses of complex regional pain syndrome.[81]

This unbalanced prominence of CRPS within workers compensation (and other types of legal claims), provides support for a conclusion that litigation/compensation is a more significant risk factor for such a diagnosis, than are health issues. Such a conclusion would also be supported by scientific findings from research that considered chronic pain claims more generally.[15,16] In addition to the scientific prominence of litigation/compensation as a risk factor for chronic pain generally, the information provided in the publications referenced above indicates that CRPS appears to be an especially good example of the role of litigation/compensation as a risk factor chronic pain.

This strong association between litigation/compensation and the CRPS construct necessitates consideration of the issues that typically emerge within relevant legal claims, or which are inherent to such legal claims.

A variety of scientific, legal, and healthcare principles are utilized in this discussion, but it can be noted at this starting point that the entire discussion is shaped by the fundamental legal and forensic principle that the plaintiff/claimant almost always has the burden of proof, thus, a claim involving complex regional pain syndrome must be proven by the claimant/plaintiff; a party defending against such a claim is not required to disprove the claim.[61,72]

Summary of the application of medical-legal considerations to claims of CRPS

When addressing legal principles and their application to medical claims, definitions are important. If the reader is unfamiliar with these definitions, a basic understanding of them can be found in an article addressing evidence based medicine causation analysis within the context of workers compensation claims by Sinclair.[73]

The remainder of this section frequently uses variations of the word "reliable". The legal use of the word "reliable" refers to a legal principle of "evidentiary reliability".[38,73] That legal principle is reportedly based on "scientific validity" --grounded in the methods and procedures of science/more than subjective belief or unsupported speculation, as well as "scientific reliability," which refers to the reproducibility of findings.[38]

The information which a doctor provides to a legal process should be sufficiently based on reliable/validated facts, reliable/validated data, and reliable/validated principles.[73] Currently, there is no scientific basis for concluding that any legal claim which involves CRPS can be deducted from reliable/validated facts, data, or principles. There are substantial obstacles to credibly concluding that a claim involving CRPS can be based on reliable/validated facts, data, or principles.

Evidentiary reliability of information which a doctor provides to a legal process can be evaluated in terms of whether the underlying theory and techniques can be scientifically tested, whether they have been tested, and whether they have survived such scientific testing.[73] In other texts, this issue has been referred to as the "testability and falsification" consideration[38] or "the refutability principle".[21] It would be difficult to conclude that there can be, or has been, credible scientific tests of the theories and techniques on which a claim of CRPS would be based. What is revealed when CRPS literature is reviewed is that there are substantial obstacles to credibly concluding relevant theories or techniques could be, or have been, scrutinized through credible scientific efforts. There are also substantial obstacles to concluding that relevant principles or techniques could survive credible scientific scrutiny.

Furthermore, the evidentiary reliability of information which a doctor provides to a legal process can be evaluated in terms of whether the error rate is known for the underlying method.[73] There is no credible basis for concluding that the error rate is known for the various modern methods that potentially produce a diagnostic claim of CRPS. In fact, modern methods in this regard, their shortcomings, and their lack of scientific testability, are discussed in Appendix A. The more detailed information reveals substantial obstacles to credibly concluding that the error rate has been established for the relevant diagnostic methods, and to credibly concluding that the error rate could be established for any of them.

A model for communicating with the legal system about claims involving CRPS

The diagnostic system for mental disorders has repeatedly been specified as a model for efforts that contributed to the creation of the diagnostic methods for CRPS.[24,39,45-47,50]

Elements of the diagnostic system for mental disorders which have been replicated in the various diagnostic methods for CRPS include: a lack of causative implications, a lack of pathophysiology, a descriptive focus rather than an explanatory or etiological focus, and a lack of scientific credibility. [6-13,19-22,35,67]

The nature of the diagnostic systems for mental disorders and CRPS has also been specifically identified as an obstacle to scientific advancement.[51] This issue indicates that the CRPS construct is lacking in scientific credibility, is actually evasive of science, and creates obstacles to the advancement of health science. In other words, the nature of CRPS is both a-scientific and anti- scientific. If the premise that health care should be scientifically credible is accepted, then the construct of CRPS has no place in health care.

Given the repeatedly documented history of the diagnostic system for mental disorders serving as a model for the modern conceptualizations of CRPS, the implications of that model should be fully manifested in regard to CRPS. For example, the diagnostic system for mental disorders has repeatedly been inextricably linked to published warnings that the system cannot be credibly used to support legal claims (such warnings have actually been placed in the various editions of the manuals for that system which have been published since the creation of CRPS).[3-5] Similar published warnings regarding CRPS have not been identified in the literature.

Such warnings are provided here (consistent with the repeatedly published reports that the modern conceptualizations of CRPS are modeled after the diagnostic system for mental disorders)

- A claim that involves the construct of CRPS does not allow for a credible legal determination (or a credible scientific determination, or even a credible clinical determination) that an individual has a health abnormality.

- A claim that involves the construct of CRPS syndrome does not allow for a credible legal determination (or a credible scientific determination, or even a credible clinical determination) that a clinical presentation has been caused by an injury, an accident, occupational issues, or any other claimed causes that are common in legal/compensation claims.

- A claim that involves the construct of CRPS does not allow for a credible legal determination (or a credible scientific determination, or even a credible clinical determination) that an individual is vocationally disabled, has work limitations, or is in need of work restrictions.

- A claim that involves the construct of CRPS does not allow for a credible legal determination (or a credible scientific determination, or even a credible clinical determination) that a clinical presentation is permanent, involves permanent impairment, warrants an impairment rating greater than zero, etc.

- The involvement of the construct of CRPS in a claim is an obstacle to credibility for any other legal determinations (and any other scientific determinations, and any other clinical determinations) that would be supportive of the legal/compensation claim.

A scientifically credible definition developed specifically for legal contexts

Early in a process in which a doctor is asked to interact with the legal system, that doctor will typically be asked to provide definitions. Consequently, this discussion of legal considerations for claims of CRPS provides definitional information.

Attorneys demonstrate a misdirected (and yet pervasive) tendency toward asking doctors to act as dictionaries. Specifically, attorneys commonly ask doctors to provide a definition immediately upon request, and based on nothing other than the doctor's memory (in spite of the notoriously unreliable nature of human memory). It is especially notable that attorneys typically request this information from doctors, even though there is no reason to suspect that a doctor will have any expertise in creating definitions, and even though the attorneys could have turned instead to readily available published definitions.

Attorneys almost always make such requests during depositions and trials, without having forewarned the doctor that the request for a definition would be made (thereby preventing the doctor from being prepared to comply with such requests). This extremely common set of circumstances makes it unfeasible for the doctor to credibly offer the requested definition. Consequently, the doctor would be wise to respond by explaining that the doctor has not been trained to serve as a dictionary, by additionally explaining that the doctor's expertise does not involve spontaneously creating definitions, and by advising the attorney to look elsewhere for such definitions (e.g., in dictionaries or other published sources which involve relevant expertise. For health science issues, the relevant expertise for such a definition would involve scientific credibility, as well as expertise in the development of definitions.

If, instead of the common scenario described above, an attorney were to request a definition in a credible fashion which actually makes it feasible for the doctor to work toward providing such a definition, then the doctor could consider complying with the request.

Specifically in regard to CRPS, regardless of the circumstance in which an attorney asks for a definition of that construct, there is not an adequate published definition. Published definitions are unreliable and contradict one another, are especially inadequate in terms of scientific credibility, and are especially inadequate for the legal contexts which dominate claims of CRPS.

Therefore, the following list is offered as definitional information which a doctor can offer to an attorney who asks the doctor to define the concept of CRPS. In the common context in which an attorney makes the non-credible request for a doctor to act as a dictionary, the doctor can advise the attorney to go read this text (unless the doctor happens to have this text at hand, and is allowed to read aloud from it).

The definitional information which is provided below is fact-based, and referenced. This distinguishes it from many other publications which supposedly provide definitions of CRPS[62,63,71,48] in that those other publications appear to be based on what someone thinks CRPS should mean, rather than being based on the actual characteristics of the construct and reporting the results of scientific findings regarding people who obtain such a diagnosis. Barriers include unreliability, high rate of involvement in legal claims, high probability the claimant will have a personality disorder and will probably demonstrate an invalid clinical presentation when tested objectively.

The list of definitional issues is long, and that length is a reflection of the unreliable, highly variable nature of the complex regional pain syndrome construct.

Complex regional pain syndrome is an unreliable concept[9,22] that was created by a "special   consensus conference" which was reportedly organized by two people in 1993.[71*]

This concept was initially formalized in the 1994 edition of the IASP's *Classification of Chronic Pain*.[62]

That initial formalization substantially strays from the later published reports of the results of the 1993 conference. For example, while the 1993 conference conceptualized a history of a "noxious event" as being a necessary part of the CRPS diagnosis[71], the IASP 1994 formalization of the construct did not require such a history.[62] This initial discrepancy highlights the unreliability which has plagued the CRPS construct from its beginning.

The IASP's initial formalization is not being included in this list of definitional information, because that initial formalization was discontinued in 2012[63] due to its demonstrated tendency to mistakenly apply the CRPS construct to clinical presentations for which the construct was known to be irrelevant.[39,47]

This was intentionally created in a fashion which the IASP's publications characterize as "purely descriptive," rather than being explanatory, etiological, or definitional.[53]

CRPS was created in a fashion that causes it to be a pervasively non-scientific, even anti-scientific, construct.

It should be noted that the primary published report regarding the creation of the construct specifies that the associated efforts involved "acknowledging a lack of scientific understanding".[71] In fact, imperviousness to scientific advancement was reportedly intentionally built into the construct. For example, the primary published report regarding the creation of the construct indicates that the construct was intentionally created in a fashion that was so ambiguous that it would be able to "stand despite any scientific findings".[71]

The creators of the construct go so far as to deliberately take an anti-scientific approach, by creating a construct that could not be scientifically scrutinized or tested. As is explained in the Foster & Huber text[38], science is ideally a process of attempting to disprove concepts. This is an aspect of science that has been strongly embraced by American legal systems.[38,73] Consequently, when CRPS was intentionally created in a fashion that does not allow for scientific scrutiny/testing and cannot withstand any scientific efforts or discoveries, such creation was anti- scientific. This aspect of the construct has previously been emphasized in literature from the American Academy of Neurology[21], which noted that CRPS is "evasive of the refutability principle".___

This anti-scientific history would justify a conclusion that the CRPS construct is not a matter of health science, and a conclusion, borrowing words from the US Supreme Court, that it is instead simply a matter of "subjective belief or unsupported speculation".[38]

The construct was actually created due to scientific failures for the previous construct of reflex sympathetic dystrophy (RSD), rather than having been created due to any scientific discoveries which were supportive of the concept of CRPS. In other words, the creation of CRPS was prompted by "ignorance"[57] rather than from scientific knowledge.

A sub-construct of CRPS, referred to as Type I, was created by the 1993 "special consensus conference" for the purpose of replacing the failed concept of reflex sympathetic dystrophy.[62,71]

By the time that the 1993 "special consensus conference" took place, the scientific failures of the reflex sympathetic dystrophy concept were so comprehensive, that it had become apparent that the concept needed to be abandoned (removed from diagnostic taxonomy).[21,53,62,71]

This history was documented in the *Third Edition* of *Bonica's Management of Pain* in the following terms:

*At least one prominent, but late-published, report (from people who reportedly were not actually involved in the conference) claims that this 1993 conference was an activity of the International Association for the Study of Pain (IASP).[40] However, the authors of this paper have had difficulty finding confirmation of that report in earlier discussions of the conference that were published directly by the IASP, and which are attributed to people who were reportedly involved in the conference.[53,71]

"In 1993, a consensus group of pain medicine experts (a special consensus workshop of the International Association for the Study of Pain) gathered with the defined task of re-evaluating the clinical syndromes of RSD and causalgia. It was agreed by this group that these disorders were characterized by controversy and confusion with regard to diagnostic criteria, pathophysiologic mechanisms, and effective therapies. Therefore, this international consensus group agreed to dismantle the terms RSD and causalgia, to admit the field's ignorance."[57]

The 1993 "special consensus conference" apparently decided that, instead of simply allowing the failed concept of reflex sympathetic dystrophy to be terminated in the absence of any replacement, they wanted to create a new concept to replace reflex sympathetic dystrophy.[71] The justification for that creation a new construct to replace the failed reflex sympathetic dystrophy construct, in spite of reviewing every publication that we can find on the subject, remains elusive.

The complex regional pain syndrome construct was deliberately created in a fashion that is extremely ambiguous, so that it would not be subject to the same types of scientific failures that doomed the concept of reflex sympathetic dystrophy.

The intentional nature of this planned ambiguity has been specified in the primary published report, which noted that the associated efforts involved a focus on creating sufficient ambiguity to ensure that the construct would "stand despite any scientific findings".[71]

Consistent with the overall effort to ensure that CRPS would be extremely vague, the 1993 "special consensus conference" designed the construct to be an ambiguous "umbrella term", rather than to represent a reliable concept.[54,71]

As part of the development of CRPS as an ambiguous "umbrella term", the construct was applied, by the 1993 "special consensus conference"[71], and subsequently by the IASP[64] to the historical concept of causalgia (as well as reflex sympathetic dystrophy). Specifically, a sub-construct of CRPS, referred to as Type II, was created reportedly for the purpose of replacing causalgia.

Adequate justification for the application of the ambiguous umbrella construct to causalgia is unsupported, despite reviewing every publication that we can find on the subject.

This issue increased the unreliability of the CRPS construct in multiple ways. First, this meant that CRPS was conceptualized from the beginning as involving at least two distinctly different clinical scenarios. Secondly, causalgia was not actually removed from the IASP's *Classification of Chronic*

Pain.[62,63] In other words, CRPS Type II was reportedly created to replace the causalgia concept, but the causalgia concept was not actually replaced.

In 2012, the IASP changed its conceptualization of CRPS. One of the many changes involved the introduction of a third sub-construct, referred to as CRPS not otherwise specified.[63] The 2012 revision of the IASP's *Classification of Chronic Pain*[63] states that this sub-construct was created for clinical presentations which only partially match up to IASP diagnostic requirements for CRPS Type I or Type II. Consequently, there is no longer any expectation that two clinical presentations which are both labeled as CRPS will have anything in common (e.g., one can involve pain in the absence of swelling or any other characteristics of CRPS, another can involve only swelling in the absence of any pain or any other characteristics of CRPS, etc.). This development drastically increased the unreliability and ambiguity that has plagued the construct since its creation.

CRPS is devoid of any pathophysiological considerations. This is clearly specified in the original IASP formalization[62], in that the "physiology" is stated as "unknown" for both Type I and Type II.

Similarly, the 2012 revision of the IASP conceptualization states: "Pathology / Unknown. In CRPS II, the pain syndrome follows a major nerve injury, but that does not explain its pathological basis."

The concept of CRPS has not been reliable from one published source of information to another, and the concept has not even been reliable over time in regard to single sources of information.

Keep in mind, the IASP has provided multiple conceptualizations over time.[62,63]

The American Medical Association has provided multiple conceptualizations over time.[23,33,69]

At all points in history, the IASP and AMA conceptualizations of the moment have always been substantially discrepant from one another.

A wide of variety of conceptualizations have been published.[2,33,48,62-65,69,71] Such published conceptualizations extensively contradict one another. Some areas of dispute include whether the construct involves a single health condition or is instead an umbrella concept, whether the construct definitionally involves the sympathetic nervous system, whether the construct definitionally involves a history of trauma/noxious event, whether relevant clinical presentations are most often associated with a history of myocardial infarction, whether the construct applies to parts of the body other than the upper extremities, and how many sub-constructs are recognized. The conflicting nature of such conceptualizations further highlights the unreliability of the diagnosis.

A 2014 "comprehensive and critical review" emphasized the unreliability of the construct.[22]

The ambiguous and unreliable nature of the CRPS (as has been discussed above) creates additional obstacles to scientific scrutiny being applied to it.

Any scientific findings that were based on the original 1994 IASP conceptualization[62] will not be relevant to any of the modern conceptualizations (because all of the modern conceptualizations are substantially different than the 1994 IASP conceptualization).

Any scientific findings based one of the modern conceptualizations will not be relevant to any of the other modern conceptualizations, because the modern conceptualizations substantially differ from one another (the modern conceptualizations are compared and contrasted in Appendix A).

The creation of the "not otherwise specified" sub-construct[63] eliminates any hope of reliability for the CRPS construct (as was discussed above, and will be further discussed below).

The original conceptualization of CRPS was created in a fashion that causes it to be an inherently non-injury-related issue. Later published reports have similarly highlighted its non-injury-related nature.

The construct has apparently always been defined as involving a clinical presentation which is disproportionate to any claimed inciting event, such as injury.[62,63] The primary published report regarding the creation of the CRPS construct specified this disproportionality as a "distinguishing characteristic".[71]

Such disproportionality is the opposite of the dose-response gradient which is characteristic of causative relationships.[61] Consequently, this "distinguishing characteristic" actually means that an injury or any other "inciting event" is not a cause of the clinical presentation.

Similarly, a 2009 review of previously published discussions (published by the entity which initially formalized the construct – the IASP), concluded that there is also a lack of reliable association between the type of claimed injury and the pattern of the clinical presentation.[54] This means that there is not a qualitative association between a relevant clinical presentation and any claimed injury (as well as there not being an association in terms of proportionality/quantitative issues).

The lack of injury-relatedness, relevant clinical presentations have been documented as developing in the absence of any claimed injury.[45,77,80,81] Such reports are of relevance to the prevention/elimination standard of causation analysis[61] which specifies that within a causative relationship, "if the exposure can be prevented or eliminated from a population, the development of the disease or condition does not occur."

Given the multiple published reports that relevant presentations occur in the absence of even a claim of injury, attempts to claim injury- relatedness for CRPS are inconsistent with the prevention/elimination standard of causation analysis. They are also inconsistent with the dose-response gradient standard).

The inherently non-injury-related nature of the CRPS is also highlighted by all of the following:

- The original IASP conceptualization specified that a history of injury (or any   other type of "noxious event") was not a required part of the construct.[62]

- Efforts to apply some minimal scientific scrutiny to that original IASP conceptualization resulted in a recommendation for the elimination of even the optional criterion which involved consideration of a history of injury (or any other type of "noxious event").[45]

- That optional 1994 IASP criterion which involved consideration of a history of injury/ "noxious event" is completely absent from modern conceptualizations.[2,63,65,69]

Scientific findings have indicated that most cases which involve a diagnosis of CRPS will be associated with a legal claim of some form (e.g., workers compensation claim or personal injury lawsuit.[1,75,81] This fact, combined with the definitional lack of association between CRPS and any pathophysiology, provides a credible basis for concluding that a diagnosis of CRPS in an individual case which involves compensation incentives is best conceptualized as an artifact of those incentives, rather than being purely conceptualized as a health issue.

Whenever this diagnosis is made, some form of pre-existing psychopathology is usually involved in the clinical presentation.

Scientific findings have revealed strong associations between relevant clinical presentations and pre-existing psychopathology, specifically including personality disorders, depressive disorders, vulnerability to anxiety, vulnerability to somatization, and fear of movement.[10,11,15,16,34,44]

While the same is true for chronic benign pain in general[15,16], scientific findings have indicated that people who develop CRPS-like presentations are even more psychologically dysfunctional than other chronic pain patients.[26]

This set of circumstances provides a credible basis for concluding that a diagnosis of CRPS in an individual case is best conceptualized as a manifestation of psychopathology (in the extremely rare case which does not involve compensation incentives), or as a consequence of the interaction of compensation incentives and psychopathology.

Scientific findings and several case reports have indicated that relevant clinical presentations are often self-inflicted.[29,32,59,68,76]

Such scientific findings are supportive of the following conclusion from the American Medical Association's *AMA Guides to the Evaluation of Disease and Injury Causation:*[75]

"Anyone who wishes to pretend to have CRPS can simulate enough 'signs' to meet point 3 in these criteria" (referring to the portion of the Budapest criteria which are mislabeled as "signs", but which are actually under the control of the patient).

Scientific findings have indicated that all of the objectively verifiable clinical issues that have been written into various conceptualizations of CRPS (e.g., swelling, trophic changes) can be created through disuse.[30]

In the American Medical Association conceptualizations of CRPS[33,69] the potential for such objective signs to be caused by disuse has been specified as the apparent link between:

- the individual's pre-existing psychology and the development of a CRPS-like presentation
- malingering and the development of a CRPS-like presentation

The concept of CRPS has not been scientifically validated as actually corresponding to any health condition.[20-22,35,67,69]

Scientific findings have indicated that relevant clinical presentations have a very favorable prognosis, typically resolving within months.[70] The majority of people who receive such a diagnosis will demonstrate invalid clinical presentations, when scientifically validated objective testing is administered.[43]

A 2014 "comprehensive and critical review" concluded that: "There are no standards which can be applied to the diagnosis and would fulfill definitions of evidence- based medicine."[22] In other words, a scientifically credible method for justifying such a diagnostic claim does not exist.

A variety of health science publications have called for the abandonment of the CRPS construct.[20-22,35,67] In addition to the construct's ambiguity, unreliability, and lack of scientific credibility, the reasons for such calls for abandonment of the construct include reports that the utilization of the construct deprives patients of adequate diagnosis, and consequently, deprives patients of adequate treatment.

CRPS does not involve neuropathic (or neurogenic) pain.

The lack of relevance of the concept of neuropathic pain for the "type one" sub-construct of CRPS has a tradition of being clearly documented by the IASP[54] and other high- profile organizations.[41]

In contrast, CRPS Type II was originally conceptualized by the IASP as involving neuropathic (or neurogenic) pain.[31]

In 2011, the IASP published a variety of publications which discussed a new definition of neuropathic pain, and the fact (resulting from that new definition of neuropathic pain) that this new definition meant that the entire construct of CRPS was now conceptualized as being "non-neuropathic".[44,55]

Historically, there have been some issues which were almost definitional for CRPS(almost common to the various conceptualizations). These issues are listed below. It should first be noted that the near-definitional nature of these issues has now been compromised by the introduction of the "not otherwise specified" sub-construct. The issues which were almost definitional prior to the introduction of the "not otherwise specified" sub-construct included:

- The concept involved a syndrome. Given a definition of "syndrome" such as "a set of symptoms that occur together," (Dorland's Illustrated Medical Dictionary, 32nd Edition) this aspect of the construct has been clearly discontinued by the introduction of the "not otherwise specified" sub-construct which eliminates the premise that this involves any set of symptoms which reliably occur together. In fact, given the variability in clinical presentations which has been allowed by the various conceptualizations of CRPS, it does not appear that the construct ever actually involved a syndrome. Literature does not support an adequate explanation for the discrepancy between the labeling of the construct as a syndrome, versus the anti-syndromic variability that has been allowed by every conceptualization of the construct.

- Prior to the introduction of "not otherwise specified" sub-construct, CRPS was a combination of subjective symptoms (e.g. pain) and signs which could be objectively verified (e.g. swelling, trophic changes). This formerly definitional issue is especially important to note, as the authors of this paper have repeatedly seen clinical presentations which involved nothing other than a complaint of pain, and yet the presentation was diagnosed as CRPS (such cases came to the attention of committee members regularly, even prior to the creation of the "not otherwise specified" sub-construct).

- Historically, CRPS has been defined by the clinical presentation being inconsistent with any claimed cause (e.g., disproportionately severe in regard to any claimed cause, anatomically inconsistent with any claimed cause, etc.).

- The "Type II" sub-construct involves a history of unambiguous injury[69] to a large[71] or major[46] peripheral[69] nerve. But, the clinical presentation was inconsistent with any such injury.

- In contrast to Type II, the "Type I" sub-construct does not involve a history of nerve injury.[69,41,54]

The phrase "*chronic* regional pain syndrome" has been used specifically for the purpose of distinguishing clinical scenarios which definitely do not involve complex regional pain syndrome, from those which supposedly do involve complex regional pain syndrome.

One of the definitional significant differences between these two issues is that conceptualizations of complex regional pain syndrome include trophic changes, while "*chronic* regional pain syndrome" refers to clinical presentations which specifically do not involve trophic changes.

The scenarios which are categorized as "*chronic* regional pain syndromes" are distinct from the concept of complex regional pain syndrome in that the former does not involve objectively verifiable differences between one side of the body and the other (e.g. such as a difference in the circumference of soft tissues for one arm versus the other, a difference in the calluses of the palms, a differences in regard to bone density, etc.).

Examples of clinical presentations which have been categorized as *chronic* regional pain syndromes (in order to distinguish them from complex regional pain syndrome) include: the effects of inappropriately extensive immobilization, movement restrictions caused by scar tissue or neuroma, or pain which serves a socially-driven purpose for the patient.

This final point is not being formally included in the above list of definitional issues, because there are not adequate published reports of relevant systematic study. This may, therefore, be one of the most important definitional issues. The authors' informal impression is: most individual case diagnoses of CRPS are not based on any of the formal/published conceptualizations or diagnostic methods. Consequently, discussion of the formal/published conceptualizations and diagnostic methods appears to be an intellectual exercise which does not apply to the overwhelming majority of cases which involve diagnostic claims of CRPS. It is highly unlikely that the work of the diagnosing doctor in an individual claim adhered to such professional standards. The true meaning of an individual claim of CRPS is probably limited to the scientific findings which have been summarized above (e.g., the patient probably has a history of involvement in legal claims, the clinical presentation probably involves psychopathology, the clinical presentation will probably be revealed to be invalid if objective testing is utilized, etc.).

Complex regional pain syndrome is not a reliable construct

As was discussed above, legal systems typically involve an expectation that information provided to that system by a doctor must be based on reliable facts and data, and that the information must be based on reliable principles.[38,73] As was discussed above, this legal issue use of the word "reliable" refers to scientific validity as well as scientific reliability. This section will focus on scientific reliability, and later sections will add scientific validity to the discussion.

In regard this legal expectation of scientific reliability, any information which a doctor might offer in support of a legal claim of CRPS should involve justification for the inherent claim that CRPS is a reliable construct. At a minimum, this would mean that the construct would have the same meaning from time to time, from case to case, and every time that it was used.

The authors are not aware of any credible justification for such a claim that the complex regional pain syndrome construct is reliable at this minimal level.

In fact, it does not actually appear possible for such a claim to be justified. There are two primary indications of the unreliability of the construct:

- The construct of CRPS has not been reliable historically (the construct has repeatedly changed over time) (e.g., American College of Occupational and Environmental Medicine 2008; Brigham 1999; Cocchiarella & Anderson 2001; Ensalada 2007; Harden & Bruehl 2005; Harden et al. 2007; Harden and Bruehl 2010a; Merskey & Bogduk 1994; Merskey & Bogduk 2012; Mosby's Medical Dictionary, 9th Edition 2013; ODG Treatment in Workers Comp; Rondinelli et al. 2009; Stanton-Hicks 1995). Since the creation of the construct of CRPS, the International Association for the Study of Pain's *Classification of Chronic Pain* has involved two different sets of conceptualizations/protocols (Merskey & Bogduk 1994; Merskey & Bogduk 2012), the American Medical Association *Guides* library has involved at least three different sets of conceptualizations/protocols (Brigham 1999; Cocchiarella & Anderson 2001; Ensalada 2007; Rondinelli et al. 2009), and additional conceptualizations have emerged from a variety of other sources (e.g., American College of Occupational and Environmental Medicine 2008; Harden & Bruehl 2005; Harden et al. 2007; Harden & Bruehl 2010a; Mosby's Medical Dictionary, 9th Edition 2013; Stanton- Hicks 1995).

- The history of unreliability continues, with multiple definitions/conceptualizations/protocols in existence currently, and the various definitions/conceptualizations/protocols involving substantial inconsistencies from one to another (e.g., American College of Occupational and Environmental Medicine 2008; Harden & Bruehl 2005; Harden et al. 2007; Harden & Bruehl 2010a; Merskey & Bogduk 2012; Mosby's Medical Dictionary, 9th Edition 2013; ODG Treatment in Workers Comp; Rondinelli et al. 2009).

A detailed discussion of the continuing unreliability of modern conceptualizations and protocols for this construct is provided in Appendix A. For example, Appendix A describes the manner in which modern conceptualizations of the construct are not consistent with one another, thereby highlighting the unreliability of the construct.

The unreliability is not limited to discrepancies between various conceptualizations. Unreliability is also demonstrated within single conceptualizations. For example, various published versions of the Budapest protocol are inconsistent with one another.[46,47] The is created that a clinical presentation which matches up to the construct of CRPS according to the 2005 report regarding inconsistencies are sufficiently substantial that the possibility the Budapest protocol, might not match up to that construct according to the 2007 report regarding that same protocol.[46,47] The 2005 and 2007 reports are supposedly documenting a single conceptualization, as each report specifies that it is documenting a conceptualization that was "adopted and codified" for purposes of "being proposed to the Committee for Classification of Chronic Pain of the IASP for inclusion in future revisions of their formal taxonomy and diagnostic criteria for pain states."[46,47] There is no explanation of the discrepancies between the 2005 and 2007 reports regarding the nature of the Budapest protocol.

Appendix A also provides a detailed discussion of the manner in which the CRPS has actually become increasingly unreliable over time. For example, the relatively recent introduction of the sub-construct "CRPS, not otherwise specified" eliminates even the slightest hint of reliability for the construct. The 2012 IASP conceptualization specifies that the "not otherwise specified" sub-construct was created so that CRPS could be applied to a clinical presentation which "partially meets CRPS criteria, not better explained by any other condition". This means, for example, that a clinical presentation that involves nothing other than an unexplained complaint of pain, or nothing other than an unexplained complaint of occasional swelling, can now be given a diagnosis of CRPS. The 2012 IASP conceptualization explains that this sub-construct was created "to capture any patients previously diagnosed with CRPS who now do not meet criteria as elaborated above," but that explanation does not mitigate the unreliability, because of issues such as the following:

- It does not require that the previous diagnosis was based on any standardized or professionally endorsed diagnostic method. Therefore, this sub-construct provides a formal justification (but not a credible justification) for a previous diagnosis of CRPS even if that diagnosis was baseless, mistaken, made by a doctor who had no actual understanding of the CRPS, etc.

- If the explanation was intended to communicate more than it actually communicates, in the form of intending to explain that the "not otherwise specified" sub-construct was created for cases that had previously been diagnosed with CRPS according to the 1994 IASP conceptualization, then it should be noted that empirical testing of the 1994 conceptualization revealed that most research participants who were diagnosable as having CRPS under that conceptualization were from the research group who were known to definitely not have a clinical presentation which corresponded to the construct.[27] Consequently, the "not otherwise specified" sub-construct would be following a historical model that was empirically demonstrated to be incorrect in most of the cases for which it produced a diagnosis of CRPS. Hopefully, it is obvious that continuing such a tradition of extreme false diagnosis is not advisable or credible: and continuing such a tradition exacerbates the unreliability that is already pervasive within the construct of CRPS.

Because of considerations such as those listed above, the emergence of this sub-construct eliminates any expectation that two separate cases which share this diagnostic label will have anything in common, and allows for a

CRPS diagnosis to be made when even the unreliable and non-validated diagnostic requirements for the other sub-constructs do not apply to the case. This raises the level of unreliability so high that a conclusion is supported that there is absolutely no reliability for the construct of CRPS.

The unreliability of the construct, as described above, prevents generalizability for any scientific findings which might emerge from scientific efforts that are focused on the construct. In other words, scientific findings that are based on one variation of the construct will not be relevant to other variations of the construct. This lack of generalizability is itself another form of unreliability, and adds another layer to the unreliable nature of the CRPS.

Another example of the continuing unreliability of the construct, and the lack of generalizability of any relevant scientific findings, involves the manner in which the 2012 IASP conceptualization[63] and the various published versions of the Budapest protocol[46,47] call for scientific investigations to use a different conceptualization and protocol than that which is used within clinical work. This calls for a set of circumstances in which scientific work will be focused on a different construct than clinical work, even though the scientific work and the clinical work will both use the same label for their different constructs. If this IASP and Budapest model is actually adopted, then scientific findings will have a lack of relevance for clinical work (because the scientific findings will be based on a different construct than that which the clinical work focuses on).

The examples of unreliability that are discussed above eliminate any hope of credibly claiming that CRPS is a reliable construct (in legal terms, a reliable fact, or a reliable principle). Consequently, only a very simple discussion is provided, in the remainder of this section, of additional examples of the unreliability.

The unreliability of the construct is perhaps even more prominent in the history of relevant scientific work than in the history of its conceptualizations. The results of two review processes have revealed that there has been a lack of reliability for the definitions and diagnostic methods that were used in relevant scientific projects.[66,78] Additionally, scientific findings regarding the construct have been so unreliable that a review of such findings, published by the organization that originally formalized the construct (the IASP), included the conclusion that the number of variations appears to be "nearly endless".[82] Needless to say, a construct that involves "nearly endless" variations cannot credibly be characterized as being reliable. Even more unreliability has been introduced since the publication of the literature that has been referenced in this paragraph, as the American Medical Association[69] , the International Association for the Study of Pain[63], the American College of Occupational and Environmental Medicine[2], and other sources have published additional definitions/protocols since those reviews were published. In fact, he 2012 IASP protocol/definition includes the "not otherwise specified" sub-construct which eliminates any hope of reliability for the construct.

Another layer of unreliably was introduced by a published discussion of CRPS as a "functional disorder".[58] That discussion has a high level of prominence because it was published directly by the organization that originally formalized the construct (the IASP), and because it was authored by the primary editor of a prominent pain management textbook.[57] That author's textbook defined "functional disorders" as pain complaints that are a variation of normal functioning (rather than being a health abnormality).[57] Such equating of CRPS with normal functioning, creates yet another level of unreliability for any attempts to claim that the construct represents a health abnormality. Consistent with such characterization of relevant presentations as a variation of normal functioning, a 2014 "comprehensive and critical review,"[22] summarized scientific findings which indicated that many of the issues which have been written into CRPS are normal after injury (including after surgery), and highlighted the manner in which the construct does not provide clear direction for determining when such issues should be categorized as pathological rather than normal.

The unreliability is so severe that it is even prominent within subtypes of CRPS syndrome (in other words, the unreliability is not limited to differences between the different subtypes). For example:

- Scientific findings have indicated that even within a given subtype, at least three distinct syndromes have been identified.[28] Such findings provide even more evidence that there is not a credible basis for claiming that CRPS will be reliable from one case to another (even sub-constructs will not be reliable from one case to another).

- As was discussed above, unreliability for the "Type II" sub-construct has been demonstrated by the discrepancy between the IASP's published reports that this sub- construct was created to replace causalgia, versus the fact that causalgia has not been replaced (causalgia has been listed in every version of the IASP's *Classification of Chronic Pain* which has included the construct of complex regional pain syndrome).[62,63]

- The "not otherwise specified" sub-construct eliminates any expectation of reliability.

This section has been largely limited to referencing some of the more prominent publications regarding CRPS, such as publications from the International Association for the Study of Pain, publications from the American Medical Association. A 2014 "comprehensive and critical review" referenced a far greater set of literature, and similarly highlighted the extreme unreliability of the construct.[22]

It cannot be credibly claimed that the construct of complex regional pain syndrome matches up to an actual health phenomenon

This section is of relevance to the scientific validity considerations that are inherent in the expectation of "evidentiary reliability" from legal systems.[38,73]

Any information which a doctor might offer within a legal context (e.g., expert witness testimony) in support of a claim of CRPS should, according to the legal principles discussed above, provide justification for the inherent claim that CRPS is an accurate characterization of an actual health condition.

There is no supporting literature for any credible justification for such a claim.

There are health science publications which contradict any such claim. Examples include publications which highlight the general lack of scientific support for the premise that the construct adequately characterizes any actual health condition, including publications which characterize it as a mythical construct that is impossible to validate.[21,22,35,67,69] At least one prominent publication indicates the construct refers to a variation of normal human functioning, rather than a health abnormality.[58]

Information that was discussed in the previous section of this report is also of relevance for this section. For example, the nature of the modern definitions/conceptualizations/protocols for CRPS allows for the label to be applied to cases which have nothing in common with one another. Therefore, it cannot be credibly claimed that that there is a discrete health condition to which this construct specifically applies.

The scientific reliability problems that were discussed above have additional relevance to this discussion of scientific validity. Specifically, a principle must be reliable before efforts can be undertaken to validate it. Efforts to validate a principle cannot be undertaken on an unreliable principle – the unreliability of the principle (in this discussion, the extreme unreliability of the construct of complex regional pain syndrome) prevents any scientific findings from applying to variations of the principle which were not directly tested in the scientific effort (a scientific test of one of the modern conceptualizations of CRPS would lack relevance for all of the other modern conceptualizations, because of the significant discrepancies between the various conceptualizations). Given the extreme unreliability of the complex regional pain syndrome construct, it does not appear possible for validity of the construct to be established (or even for credible attempts to establish validity to be undertaken).

There is no reliable or scientifically credible method for justifying a diagnosis of   complex   regional pain syndrome

This section is also of relevance to the scientific validity considerations that are inherent in the expectation of "evidentiary reliability" from legal systems.[38,73]

A doctor who offers support for a legal claim involving CRPS should provide justification for the inherent claim that a scientifically validated method exists for establishing that diagnosis in an individual case.

Try to locate a credible justification for such a claim....it does not exist. In other words, there is no credible scientific validation for any of the diagnostic methods/protocols for CRPS. Instead, scientific publications explain a credible method for justifying a diagnostic claim of complex regional pain syndrome does not exist, and that the construct is of a nature which will prevent the development of a credible method for making such a diagnosis.[20-22]

Information which indicates that no such validated method is available includes that which comes from publications regarding the unreliable method referred to as the Budapest protocol. This appears to be the modern method which has been subjected to the most extensive quasi-scientific scrutiny (the relevant publications reveal that such attempted scrutiny has been of a minimal nature, even though it has been more extensive than the scientific efforts undertaken in response to any other modern method). The unreliability of this protocol (it takes different forms in different publications), and its lack of validity, are discussed in greater detail in Appendix A and in other chapters. This section provides just a few highlights from those more detailed discussions.

The relevant publications reveal that the investigations that have been undertaken in regard to the unreliable Budapest protocol have not been of a nature that could actually provide validation for that protocol.[22] For example:

- The documented investigations have misused the concepts of specificity and sensitivity, by applying them to an issue (complex regional pain syndrome) which does not correspond to an actual health condition that can be objectively verified in any individual case.

- The inadequacy of such efforts was actually indicated in the introduction for the book which provided the first published discussion of that protocol stating, "It is common to talk about the sensitivity and specificity of tests and diagnostic criteria for the establishment of a diagnosis. This is only meaningful, however, if there is a gold standard to determine that the disease is present. For CRPS, we have no such gold standard. Until we develop some type of test, or constellation of signs and symptoms that are unique to this entity, we cannot determine the reliability of any diagnostic criterion."[58] It is suspected that this passage was actually referring to validity when the word "reliability" was used, because the lack of a gold standard for objectively establishing the presence of a health condition which matches CRPS indeed prevents the development of scientific validity for any diagnostic method (and prevents meaningful use of concepts such as sensitivity, specificity, positive predictive value, negative predictive value, and diagnostic accuracy).

- Consequently, the "scientific" efforts to validate the Budapest protocol are actually quasi- scientific exercises in which the protocol/method is tested against whether someone thinks that a clinical presentation involves CRPS, rather than the method being tested against whether a clinical presentation actually involves CRPS. Such exercises are essentially meaningless.

This misdirected history of flawed claims of validation for some variation of the Budapest protocol is discussed in greater detail in Appendix A and within other chapters.

Finally, it can be noted that scientific findings have indicated that components which are common to almost all modern methods (physical examination findings involving temperature, swelling, etc.) are not reliable.[36,79] Such unreliability prevents the establishment of validity for the diagnostic methods which are built upon such components.

The premise that complex regional pain syndrome is an injury-related, work-related, accident-related, etc., phenomenon is not reliable/credible

As was discussed in detail above...

- The historical conceptualizations of CRPS (specifically including most modern conceptualizations) have been of a nature that causes CRPS to be an inherently non-injury-related, non-work-related, and non- accident-related concept.

- Multiple published reports of relevant clinical presentations developing in the absence of even a claimed injury further highlight the non-injury-related nature of CRPS.

- An IASP-published review specified that the relevant clinical presentations lack qualitative correlation with claimed injuries (as well as lacking quantitative proportionality).

This set of circumstances has been addressed in each edition of the AMA's *Guides to the Evaluation of Disease and Injury Causation*. In the first edition[60], CRPS was specified as a primary example of non-work-related issues which have been inappropriately imposed on the workers' compensation system. The text also explains that CRPS does not correspond to any disease, but instead involves a constellation of complaints that have no known cause (thereby contradicting any claims that it was caused by injury, work, an accident, etc.). The second edition[61] highlighted the strong association between such diagnoses and litigation/compensation, and addressed obstacles to credibly claiming work-relatedness, injury-relatedness, or accident-relatedness, such as the conflict between the disproportionality that is inherent in the complex regional pain syndrome construct versus the proportionality that characterizes the causative relationships. The following passages from the second edition are offered as examples:

- "CRPS cases are rare enough that no quality literature exists to provide relative risk or hazard ratio statistics. The events these patients allege as being associated with the condition do not explain the unknown pathophysiology of their illness and are not consistent with the known biology of humans healing after exposure(s)."

- "The clustering of these cases in compensation settings is problematic for considering this a physical injury in disputed cases."

The inherent lack of injury-relatedness, work-relatedness, or accident-relatedness for CRPS has been softened by the introduction of the "not otherwise specified" sub-construct. Specifically, that sub-construct does not mandate the historical definitional issue of a clinical presentation that is inconsistent with any claimed inciting event. The extreme ambiguity of the sub-construct does mean that the overall construct still fails to comply with the prevention/elimination standard of causation analysis. The extreme ambiguity of the "not otherwise specified" sub-construct causes such a diagnosis to be essentially meaningless, and thereby prevents such a diagnosis as serving as a credible basis for a claim of injury-relatedness, work-relatedness, accident-relatedness, etc. The meaninglessness of the "not otherwise specified" sub-construct calls for adamant application of the testability/falsification/refutability principles that were discussed earlier in this chapter.

Obstacles to credibly claiming injury-relatedness, work-relatedness, or accident-relatedness, for a case involving a diagnosis of CRPS also become evident when the normal method for evaluating such claims is applied. For example, the first step of the normal method[14,17,42,56,60,61,73] involves definitively establishing an explanatory diagnosis, through a method that has been scientifically validated, and based primarily on objective findings. CRPS is not capable of satisfying the requirements of this first step of the method. Relevant examples of the manner in which a diagnosis of CRPS cannot satisfy these requirements include:

- For CRPS, any such diagnosis is not going to be definitive due to the lack of scientific justification of the premise that this construct matches up to an actual health condition, the ambiguity of the construct, the unreliability of the construct, and the descriptive nature of the construct.

- Additionally, any such diagnosis is not explanatory (for the same reasons that it is not definitive).

- There is no scientifically validated diagnostic method for CRPS.

- The diagnostic methods (see Appendix A) are not primarily based on objective findings, they are instead primarily based on the subjective complaints of the examinee, and the subjective impressions of the examiner. As has been explained in the American Medical Association's *AMA Guides to the Evaluation of Disease and Injury Causation*[61] even diagnostic criteria which are labeled as "signs" within modern conceptualizations are not actually signs, but are instead based on the subjective reports of and subjective demonstrations from the examinee (as well as subjective and unreliable impressions of the examiner). Consequently, the modern conceptualizations falsely imply objectivity by labeling subjective phenomena as "signs". In fact, one of the primary promoters of the various forms of the Budapest protocol has published the observation that the protocol "forces a very heavy reliance on the subjective--the subjective response of the patient AND the subjective impression of the clinician. This is very problematic scientifically and statistically."[49]

The normal method for evaluating claims of injury-relatedness, work-relatedness, or accident- relatedness specifies that there is no need to consider the remaining steps of the method, when the first step cannot be concluded in a manner that provides preliminary support for a causation claim. Therefore, there is no need for the remaining steps of the method to be addressed in the current discussion. However, steps two through five are being discussed briefly because such discussion adds valuable information.

The key issue for the second step: In order for a causative relationship between a definitively established diagnosis and a suspected cause to be claimed in a credible fashion, the claim must be based on credible and reliable scientific findings that have convincingly established that such a specific causative link actually exists. There are no such scientific findings. It is unlikely that any such scientific findings could come into existence ---- the rules of scientific causation analysis would have to change first.

A key issue for the third step: What evidence, predominantly objective, is available that clearly verifies that the exposure to the claimed cause was of sufficient magnitude to account for the development of the claimed clinical presentation? There are no findings which reveal what level of exposure to any claimed cause is necessary in order to cause a CRPS-like presentation. Instead, we are aware of issues which indicate that this step cannot be completed in a manner which credibly supports a causation claim that is based on a diagnosis of CRPS. Such issues include the definitional disproportionality of the CRPS construct creates an obstacle to the third step being completed in a fashion that could credibly support such a causation claim. Because of that definitional issue, it appears to be impossible for scientific findings to emerge which would provide information regarding the level of exposure to any claimed cause that is necessary to cause a relevant clinical presentation (because the definitional disproportionality means that there cannot be an identifiable level of exposure – in that an identified level of exposure would imply proportionality, which would mean that the CRPS construct would not actually apply to the clinical presentation).

The published reports of relevant clinical presentations developing spontaneously (in the absence of even a claimed injury or any other claimed cause) indicates that such presentations can develop in the complete absence of any exposure to injury, workplace circumstances, accidents, or other claimed causes that are common within legal claims. This set of circumstances highlights the misdirected nature any scientific efforts to establish the necessary level of exposure to any causes that are commonly claimed by legal claimants/plaintiffs. It can be noted that such scientific efforts might not be misdirected if they were instead focused on potential risk factors which already have scientific support, and which are not typically claimed by legal claimants/plaintiffs including: disuse, narcotic medications, and psychopathology.[10,11]

The purpose of the fourth step is to consider the relevance of scientific findings for causation of the claimed clinical presentation, with an emphasis on risk factors other than the claimed cause in the case at hand. In other words, this step is dedicated to determining if other risk factors provide a better explanation for the clinical presentation than the explanation that is provided by the claimed cause. While complex regional pain syndrome was created in a fashion that causes it to be inherently non-injury-related, non-work-related, non-accident-related, etc., and while scientific findings have not been credibly supportive of such causation claims, a wide variety of other risk factors have been scientifically established for such presentations and diagnoses (See Section 5). The wealth of established non-injury-related, non-work-related, non-accident-related, etc., risk factors for such presentations and diagnoses creates obstacles to completing the fourth step in a manner that would be supportive of the common types of causation claims that are made in legal claims that involve complex regional pain syndrome.

The fifth step calls for intense scrutiny of the evidence from the individual case. One of the main issues for this step is the adequacy of the professional services that are documented or have otherwise taken plane within the case. Key questions in this regard include:

- Have other clinicians offered opinions that lack scientific credibility?

- Have clinical services been relied upon that lack scientific credibility?

It is clear that any time a clinician offers a diagnosis of complex regional pain syndrome, that clinician is offering an opinion that lacks scientific credibility (since the diagnostic construct itself lacks scientific credibility). Similarly, if the clinical services utilized any of the diagnostic methods that have been published for complex regional pain syndrome, then those services also lack scientific credibility (due to the lack of scientific validation for all of the diagnostic methods).

Complex regional pain syndrome cannot credibly serve as a basis for endorsing claims of vocational disability

When the normal method for evaluating a claim of vocational disability[74] is applied to claims that are based on a diagnosis of CRPS, substantial obstacles to credibly endorsing the disability claim become obvious. For example:

- The construct of CRPS is focused primarily on pain, and more generally involves issues that are dominated by subjective symptoms (rather than objective signs). According to the normal method for evaluating disability claims, pain and other subjective symptoms are not a credible basis for endorsing a claim of vocational disability.

- The normal method for evaluating claims of disability involves a focus on objectively identifying pathophysiology, but the construct of CRPS was intentionally created in a fashion that avoids the inclusion of any pathophysiology.[71] This means that there will not be any relevant pathophysiology which can be objectively identified in the context of such a claim. If disabling pathophysiology (or any explanatory pathophysiology) is actually identified, then the construct of CRPS does not actually apply to the case (by definition).

- As has been referenced above, scientific findings have indicated that relevant presentations typically resolve spontaneously, thereby creating an obstacle to claiming permanent disability.

- In order to be credible, any work restrictions which might be imposed on an individual who has been given this diagnosis must be based on credible scientific findings or a major consensus statement which indicates that there is a significant risk of substantial harm associated with the diagnosed individual engaging in the restricted activity. We have not found such scientific findings or statement. Instead, there is a wealth of scientific findings and statements which indicate that work would probably be beneficial for the health of any such individual.[74]

Legal claims often involve doctors being asked to create ratings of permanent impairment. Readers are first reminded of the well-documented lack of scientific credibility for the concept of impairment ratings.[69] Doctors are often faced with practical dilemmas such as the non-scientific method as it is applied to impairment ratings. If they see a need to engage in such methods, then the documentation they create for such efforts should emphasize the lack of scientific credibility, and explain the reasons why the doctor engaged in the method (such as a legal mandate).

The *AMA Guides to the Evaluation of Permanent Impairment, Sixth Edition* has a very specific advantage over prior editions in regard to the construct of workers compensation related CRPS. Specifically, the diagnostic methodology for CRPS which is delineated in that *Guides* involves a far more extensive discussion and a far more credible approach than any of the other modern methodologies (as is discussed in detail in Appendix A).

Such probable establishment of a more credible diagnosis will be in keeping with the many published reports indicating that a diagnosis of CRPS is directed, an indication of inadequate diagnostic work, harmful for the patient, and consequently should be avoided. The identification of a more credible diagnosis will have implications beyond impairment rating – it will hopefully lead to a more credible treatment plan (more credible than any that could have been based on a diagnosis of CRPS) and a better outcome, (such as minimizing the risk of any impairment actually being permanent).

If legal mandates require the use of a process for the evaluation of permanent impairment, the evaluating doctor should still consider using the diagnostic method that is delineated in the 2009 edition of the American Medical Association's impairment *Guides*. However, given the difficulties with scientific validity and the preponderance of claim behavior that this diagnosis dictates, the next section of this paper describes an alternative methodology for consideration.

Finally, readers are reminded that scientific findings have not been supportive of the premise that permanent impairment is a likely outcome for such clinical presentations.[70]

Section 7 References

1. Allen G, Galer BS, Schwartz L. Epidemiology of complex regional pain syndrome: a retrospective chart review of 134 patients. Pain. 1999; 80 (3); 539-544.

2. American College of Occupational and Environmental Medicine. Chronic Pain (Revised 2008), In: *Occupational Medicine Practice Guidelines, 2nd Edition*. American College of Occupational and Environmental Medicine, 2008.

3. American Psychiatric Association: *Diagnostic and Statistical Manual of Mental Disorders. Fourth Edition*. Washington, DC: American Psychiatric Association, 1994.

4. American Psychiatric Association: *Diagnostic and Statistical Manual of Mental Disorders. Fourth Edition - Text Revision*. Washington, DC: American Psychiatric Association, 2000.

5. American Psychiatric Association: *Diagnostic and Statistical Manual of Mental Disorders. Fifth Edition*. Washington, DC: American Psychiatric Association, 2013.

6. Barth, RJ. (2003). Complex Regional Pain Syndrome Type 1 – Obstacles to Acceptance as an Occupational Medicine Entity. The Occupational and Environmental Medicine Report, 17, 10, October, 69-76.

7. Barth, RJ, and Bohr, TW. Challenges in the IASP's Diagnostic Conceptualization for CRPS-1, Part 1. *The Guides Newsletter.* January/February, 2006a. American Medical Association.

8. Barth, RJ, and Bohr, TW. Challenges in the IASP's Diagnostic Conceptualization for CRPS-1, Part 2. *The Guides Newsletter.* March/April, 2006b. American Medical Association.

9. Barth, RJ. Complex Regional Pain Syndrome (CRPS): Unratable through the Pain Chapter. *The Guides Newsletter.* July/August, 2006c. American Medical Association.

10. Barth RJ and Haralson R. Differential Diagnosis for Complex Regional Pain Syndrome. *The Guides Newsletter,* September/October 2007a. American Medical Association.

11. Barth RJ and Haralson R. Differential Diagnosis for Complex Regional Pain Syndrome. In: Melhorn JM and Shields NN. *9th Annual Occupational Orthopaedics and Workers Compensation: A Multidisciplinary Perspective.* 2007b. American Academy of Orthopaedic Surgeons.

12. Barth RJ. A Historical Review of CRPS in The American Medical Association's Guides   Library. *The Guides Newsletter,* November/December, 2009. American Medical Association.

13. Barth RJ. A Historical Review of CRPS in The American Medical Association's Guides Library. In: Melhorn JM and Talmage JB. *13th Annual American Academy of Orthopaedic Surgeons Occupational Orthopaedics and Workers Compensation: A Multidisciplinary Perspective.* 2011. American Academy of Orthopaedic Surgeons.

14. Barth RJ. Determining Injury-Relatedness, Work-Relatedness, and Claim-Relatedness. *AMA Guides Newsletter,* May/June 2012. American Medical Association.

15. Barth RJ. Chronic Pain: Fundamental Scientific Considerations, Specifically for Legal Claims. *AMA Guides Newsletter,* Jan/Feb 2013a. American Medical Association.

16. Barth RJ. Chronic Pain: Fundamental Scientific Considerations, Specifically For Legal Claims. In: Melhorn JM (editor). *15th Annual American Academy of Orthopaedic Surgeons Occupational Orthopaedics and Workers Compensation: A Multidisciplinary Perspective.* 2013b. American Academy of Orthopaedic Surgeons.

17. Barth RJ. Determining Injury-Relatedness, Work-Relatedness, Claim-Relatedness, Etc., for All Types of Claims. Chapter N In: Melhorn JM (editor). *15th Annual American Academy of Orthopaedic Surgeons Occupational Orthopaedics and Workers Compensation: A Multidisciplinary Perspective.* 2013c. American Academy of Orthopaedic Surgeons.

18. Barth RJ (with contributions from Frances A, Kertay L, and Steinberg JS). Mental Illness: Causation Considerations Specifically for Legal Claims. Chapter 20 in: Melhorn JM (editor). *15th Annual American Academy of Orthopaedic Surgeons Occupational Orthopaedics and Workers Compensation: A Multidisciplinary Perspective.* 2013d. American Academy of Orthopaedic Surgeons.

19. Barth RJ (with contributions from Kertay L and Steinberg JS). Mental Illness. Chapter 16 in: Melhorn, JM, et al. (editors). *Guides to the Evaluation of Disease and Injury Causation, Second Edition.* 2014. American Medical Association.

20. Bass C. Complex regional pain syndrome medicalises limb pain. British Medical Journal. 2014 Apr 28;348:g2631.

21. Biller, J (Chair), et al. Neuropathic pain and Iatrogenesis. Pages 91-104 in: Iatrogenic Neurology, Continuum, 7, 2, 2001. American Academy of Neurology.

22. Borchers AT, Gershwin ME. Complex regional pain syndrome: a comprehensive and critical review. Autoimmun Rev. 2014 Mar;13(3):242-65.

23. Brigham CR (editor). *The Guides Casebook.* American Medical Association, 1999.

24. Bruehl, S., Harden, R.N., Galer, B. and Backonja, M., Factor analysis of signs and symptoms of Complex Regional Pain Syndrome: a partial validation of IASP diagnostic criteria and suggestions for change. *Neurology,* 50 (Suppl. 4) (1998) A254.

25. Bruehl S, Harden RN, Galer BS, Saltz S, Bertram M, Backonja M, Gayles R, Rudin N, Bhugra MK, Stanton-Hicks M. External validation of IASP diagnostic criteria for Complex Regional Pain Syndrome and proposed research diagnostic criteria. *Pain.* 1999 May;81(1-2):147-54.

26. Bruehl S, Husfeldt B, Lubenow TR, et al. Psychological differences between reflex sympathetic dystrophy and non-RSD chronic pain patients. *Pain,* 67 (1996) 107-114.

27. Bruehl S., Harden RN, Bradley S. Galer BS, et. al. External validation of IASP diagnostic criteria for Complex Regional Pain Syndrome and proposed research diagnostic criteria. *Pain*. 1999 May;81(1-2):147-54.

28. Bruehl S, Harden RN, Galer BS, Saltz S, Backonja M, Stanton-Hicks M. Complex regional pain syndrome: are there distinct subtypes and sequential stages of the syndrome? *Pain*. 2002 Jan;95(1-2):119-24.

29. Buijs EJ, Klijn FA, Lindeman E, van Wijck AJ. Reflex sympathetic dystrophy vs. a factitious disorder. Ned Tijdschr Geneeskd. 2000 Aug 19;144(34):1617-20.

30. Butler SH: Disuse and CRPS, in Harden RN, Baron R, Janig W (Eds): *Complex Regional Pain Syndrome*. Seattle, WA: IASP Press, 2001, pp 141-150.

31. Charlton JE (Editor). Core Curriculum for Professional Education in Pain, Third Edition. International Association for the Study of Pain. 2005.

32. Chevalier X, Claudepierre P, Larget-Piet B, & Lejonc JL. Munchhausen's syndrome simulating reflex sympathetic dystrophy. J of Rheumatol. 1996 June; 23 (6): 1111-2.

33. Cocchiarella, L. and Andersson, G. (editors) (2001). *Guides to the Evaluation of Permanent Impairment, Fifth Edition.* American Medical Association.

34. De Jong JR, Vlaeyen JWS, Onghena P, et. al. Reduction of pain-related fear in complex regional pain syndrome type I: The application of graded exposure in vivo. Pain 2005;116:264-275.

35. Del Piñal F. Editorial. I have a dream ... reflex sympathetic dystrophy (RSD or Complex Regional Pain Syndrome - CRPS I) does not exist. J Hand Surg Eur Vol. 2013 Jul;38(6):595-7.

36. Dijkstra PU, van der Schans CP, Geertzen JH. Risk perception of developing complex regional pain syndrome-1. Clin Rehabil 2003 ;17(4):944-6.

37. Ensalada LH. The Challenge of Evaluating RSD Impairment and Disability (Part 1). Guides Newsletter, November/December, 1997. Pages 3-5.

38. Foster KR & Huber PW. *Judging Science, Scientific Knowledge and the Federal Courts.* The MIT Press, 1999.

39. Galer BS, Bruehl S, Harden RN. IASP diagnostic criteria for Complex Regional Pain Syndrome: a preliminary empirical validation study. Clin J Pain 1998; 14:48-54.

40. Galer BS, Schwartz L, & Allen RJ. Complex regional pain syndromes – Type 1: Reflex Sympathetic Dystrophy and Type II: Causalgia. Chapter 20 in: Loeser JD, Butler SH, Chapman CR, & Turk DC (editors). Bonica's Management of Pain, Third Edition. Lippincott, Williams, and Wilkins, 2001.

41. Gilron I, et al. Neuropathic pain: A practical guide for the clinician. *CMAJ,* August 1, 2006, 175 (3), 265-275).

42. Glass LS, Blais BR, Genovese E, et al. (editors). Occupational Medicine Practice Guidelines, Second Edition. OEM Press, 2004.

43. Greiffenstein M, Gervais R, Baker WJ, Artiola L, Smith H. Symptom validity testing in medically unexplained pain: a chronic regional pain syndrome type 1 case series. The Clinical Psychologist. 2013;27(1):138-47.

44. Haanpää M1, Attal N, Backonja M, et al. NeuPSIG guidelines on neuropathic pain assessment. Pain. 2011 Jan;152(1):14-27.

45. Harden RN, Bruehl S, Galer BS, et al. Complex regional pain syndrome: are the IASP diagnostic criteria valid and sufficiently comprehensive? *Pain,* 83 (1999), 211-219.

46. Harden RN & Bruehl S. Diagnostic Criteria: The Statistical Derivation of the Four Criterion Factors. Chapter 4 in: Wilson PR, Stanton-Hicks M, & Harden RN (editors). *CRPS: Current Diagnosis and Therapy.* IASP Press, Seattle, 2005.

47. Harden RN, Bruehl S, Stanton-Hicks M, Wilson PR. Proposed new diagnostic criteria for complex regional pain syndrome. Pain Med. 2007 May-Jun;8(4):326-31.

48. Harden RN & Bruehl S. Complex Regional Pain Syndrome. Chapter 25 in: Fishman SM, Ballantyne JC, & Rathmell JP (editors). *Bonica's Management of Pain, Fourth Edition.* Lippincott Williams & Wilkins, 2010a.

49. Harden RN. Objectification of the diagnostic criteria for CRPS. Pain Med. 2010b Aug;11(8):1212-5.

50. Harden RN. The Diagnosis of CRPS: Are we there yet? PAIN, 153 (2012) 1142–143. Hay BL. Allocating the Burden of Proof. Indiana Law Journal, 72, 3, p.651-679, 1997. Huyghe I, Carp L, De BP, Driessens M, Block P: Self-induced hypoxia to mimic the clinical symptoms of reflex sympathetic dystrophy. *Clin Nucl Med.* 2002;27:48-49.

51. Insel T. Transforming Diagnosis. NIMH Director's Blog. April 29, 2013. http://www.nimh.nih.gov/about/director/2013/transforming-diagnosis.shtml. Accessed July 11, 2014.

52. Janig W, Blumberg H, Boas RA, & Campbell JA. The reflex sympathetic dystrophy syndrome: consensus statement and general recommendations for diagnosis and clinical research. In: Bond MR, Charlton JE, & Woolf CJ (editors). *Proceedings of the Sixth World Congress on Pain, Pain Research and Clinical Management, Volume 4,* Elsevier, Amsterdam, 1991, pages 372-375.

53. Janig W. The Puzzle of Reflex Sympathetic Dystrophy: Mechanisms, Hypotheses, Open Questions. Chapter 1 in: Janig W & Stanton-Hicks M (editors). *Reflex Sympathetic Dystrophy: A Reappraisal.* IASP Press, 1996.

54. Janig W. Autonomic Nervous System Dysfunction. Chapter 13 in: Mayer EA & Bushnell MC. Functional Pain Syndromes. IASP Press, 2009.

55. Jensen TS, Baron R, Haanpää M, et.al. A new definition of neuropathic pain. Pain. 2011 Oct;152(10):2204-5.

56. Kusnetz S, Hutchison M, eds. A Guide to the Work-Relatedness of Disease. Centers for Disease Control and Prevention; 1979. NIOSH publication 79–116.

57. Loeser JD (editor). *Bonica's Management of Pain, Third Edition.* Lippincott, Williams, and Wilkins, 2001.

58. Loeser JD. Introduction. In: Wilson PR, Stanton-Hicks M, Harden RN (editors). *CRPS: Current Diagnosis and Therapy.* International Association for the Study of Pain Press, 2005.

59. Mailis-Gagnon A, Nicholson K, Blumberger D, Zurowski M. Characteristics and period prevalence of self-induced disorder in patients referred to a pain clinic with the diagnosis of complex regional pain syndrome. *Clin J Pain.* 2008 Feb;24(2):176-85.

60. Melhorn JM and Ackerman WE (editors). *Guides to the Evaluation of Disease and Injury Causation.* American Medical Association, 2008.

61. Melhorn JM, Talmage JB, Ackerman WE, & Hyman MH (editors). *AMA Guides to the Evaluation of Disease and Injury Causation, Second Edition.* American Medical Association, 2014.

62. Mersky H, Bogduk N (Eds): *Classification of Chronic Pain, Second Edition.* Seattle,WA: IASP Press, 1994.

63. Merskey H, & Bogduk N (editors). *Classification of Chronic Pain, Second Edition (Revised).* International Association for the Study of Pain, 2012.

64. *Mosby's Medical Dictionary, Ninth Edition.* Elsevier, 2013.

65. *ODG Treatment in Workers Comp*: http://www.odg-twc.com/ Accessed July 11, 2014.

66. Reinders MF, Geertzen JH, Dijkstra PU. Complex regional pain syndrome type I: use of the International Association for the Study of Pain diagnostic criteria defined in 1994. *Clin J Pain.* 2002 Jul-Aug;18(4):207-15.

67. Ring D, Barth R, and Barsky A. Evidence-based medicine: disproportionate pain and disability, *Journal of Hand Surgery*, volume 34a, August 2010, 1345-1347.

68. Rodriguez-Moreno J, Ruiz-Martin J. M., Mateo-Soria L., et al. Munchhausen's syndrome simulating reflex sympathetic dystrophy. *Annals of Rheumatic Diseases.* 1990; 49: 1010-1012.

69. Rondinelli RD, Brigham CR, Genovese E, et al. (Editors). *Guides to the Evaluation of Permanent Impairment Sixth Edition (Second Printing).* American Medical Association, 2009.

70. Sandroni P, Benrud-Larson LM, McClelland RL, and Low PA. Complex regional pain syndrome, type I: incidence in Olmsted County, a population-based study. *Pain* 2003; 103: 199-207.

71. Stanton-Hicks M, Janig W, Hassenbusch S, Haddox JD, Boas R, Wilson P. Reflex sympathetic dystrophy: changing concepts and taxonomy. *Pain.* 1995; 63:127-133.

72. Simon RI (editor). Posttraumatic Stress Disorder in Litigation, Guidelines for Forensic Practice, Second Edition. American Psychiatric Publishing, Inc. 2003.

73. Sinclair DC. Epidemiology in the Courtroom: An Evidence-Based Paradigm for the Determination of Causation in Compensation Environments. *Journal of Occupational Medicine,* 52, Number 4, April 2010, pages 456-461.

74. Talmage JB, Melhorn JM, & Hyman MH. AMA Guides to the Evaluation of Work Ability and Return to Work, Second Edition. American Medical Association, 2011.

75. Talmage JB, Melhorn JM, Ackerman WE, & Barth RJ. Musculoskeletal Disorders: Conditions of Uncertain Pathophysiology – Acute and Chronic Pain, in: Melhorn, JM, et al. (editors). *Guides to the Evaluation of Disease and Injury Causation, Second Edition.* 2014. American Medical Association.

76. Taskaynatan MA, Balaban B, Karlidere T, Ozgul A, Tan AK, Kalyon TA. Factitious disorders encountered in patients with the diagnosis of reflex sympathetic dystrophy. *Clin Rheumatol.* 2005 Sep;24(5):521-6.

77. Veldman PH, et al. Signs and symptoms of reflex sympathetic dystrophy: Prospective study of 829 patients. *Lancet*, 1993, 342 (8878): 1012-6.

78. van de Beek WJ, Schwartzman RJ, van Nes SI, Delhaas EM, van Hilten JJ. Diagnostic criteria used in studies of reflex sympathetic dystrophy. Neurology. 2002 Feb 26;58(4):522-6.

79. van de Vusse AC, Stomp-van den Berg SG, de Vet HC, Weber WE. Interobserver reliability of diagnosis in patients with complex regional pain syndrome. Eur J Pain. 2003;7(3):259-65.

80. Van Leare M & Claessens M. The treatment of reflex sympathetic dystrophy syndrome: current concepts. *Acta Orthopaedica Belgica*, volume 58 -- supplement one -- 1992.

81. Verdugo RJ and Ochoa JL. Abnormal movements in complex regional pain syndrome: assessment of their nature. Muscle & Nerve. 2000; 23 (2), 198-205.

82. Wilson PR and Bogduk N. Retrospection, science and epidemiology of CRPS. Chapter 3 in: Wilson PR, Stanton-Hicks M, Harden RN (editors). *CRPS: Current Diagnosis and Therapy*. International Association for the Study of Pain Press, 2005.

Section 8

Impairment Ratings

The philosophy regarding impairment rating determinations for patients labeled with CRPS has been described as an enigma. On the one hand, advocates argue that this is a condition that rarely, if ever, exists, and consider the systematic approaches espoused in the American Medical Association Guides to the Evaluation of Permanent Impairment, Editions 5 and 6 to be inherently flawed. On the other hand, supporters of the legitimacy of the condition argue that the derivation of impairment ratings is correctly categorized by proper use of either the upper or lower extremity chapters and its sections that describe the approaches to those ratings. Regardless, there can be no question that the derivation of a rating process in the AMA Guides for CRPS can be loosely traced and matched to the evolution of the development of the entity known as CRPS by medical committees and groups that are described in other parts of this paper.

In an AMA Guides Newsletter article in late 2009, Barth describes the history of introduction of the term CRPS within the various AMA Guides publications.[1] Given that the term CRPS was not created until 1994[2], it does not appear within the AMA Guides to the Evaluation of Permanent Impairment until the 5th and 6th editions. Given the AMA Guides focus upon objective finding establishment serving as the underpinning for an impairment rating determination[3-6], the concept of CRPS becomes problematic. In a syndrome that has inconsistency regarding history, physical examination, and stability,[7] the mere determination of maximum medical improvement (MMI) which forms the universal state upon which impairment ratings are proffered, is legitimately argued.

When crafting an impairment rating methodology where science is weak or does not exist, the default "consensus derived" processes demand that there is at least some fundamental pre-determined basis for the argument of the methodology of impairment rating determination[6]. All editions of the Guides have taken the perspective that pain is traditionally taken into account for most organ system based impairment determination paradigms[3-6]. Given that the historical viewpoint that CRPS has been primarily driven by the presence of disproportionate pain, the syndrome in and of itself is contradictory to the Guides philosophy. Yet, for reasons that are not explained, the authors of the

5th and 6th editions elected to give CRPS its own section, its own methodology and curiously placed a pain syndrome not in the respective editions' Pain Chapter, but rather in the Upper and Lower Extremity Chapters that include musculoskeletal calamities[5-6].

Is there science behind the impairment rating process within the various editions of the AMA Guides? When reviewing the 3rd edition revised through the 6th edition (we have elected to focus only upon the 3rd edition revised and the editions of the Guides published thereafter mainly because of the fact that state worker's compensation systems do not use any editions published prior to this), the initial description of the now defunct diagnoses of causalgia and reflex sympathetic dystrophy reference very few articles[3-4]. Furthermore, these articles focus more-so upon the treatment of the condition rather than impact upon activities of daily living. In the 5th and 6th edition, references cited regarding CRPS again focus upon diagnosis and treatment as opposed to ADL impact[5-6].

What then makes CRPS (or RSD or causalgia) unique within the AMA Guides?

This is a legitimately debated question.

To arbitrarily manifest a notion that CRPS is automatically more significant regarding the diagnosis' impact upon ADLs is rather presumptuous, if indeed, we are to be considerate of the general parameters of the AMA Guides when evaluating the significance of the difference between impairment and disability.

Let us review the evolution of the impairment rating approach across the various editions.

In the 3rd edition revised, the concept of causalgia is barely mentioned. Page 41 of the text declares that "the pain associated with peripheral spinal nerve impairment, and particularly that of the median nerve, sometimes has a constant burning quality. This pain is described as a major or a minor causalgia in accordance with its severity, and it is evaluated on the same basis as other types of pain." Therefore, in the 3rd edition revised, any type of reflex sympathetic dystrophy, where there is no specific nerve injury is specifically excluded.

The text goes on to explain that the impairment rating for causalgia is determined by identification of the nerve distribution involved and grading its severity in terms of sensory involvement and multiplying the maximum impairment rating percentage for the nerve by the percent modifier assigned. The text includes an italicized admonition that "complaints of pain that cannot be characterized as above are not considered to be within the scope of this section." An important distinction in the 3rd edition revised is that there is no discussion regarding measuring joints for loss of range of motion when evaluating causalgia. Some have speculated that this may have been an oversight[8-9].

In the 4th edition, confusion is created as the text uses the terms causalgia and reflex sympathetic dystrophy interchangeably. Given that the 4th edition was published in 1993, this is illustrative of the "chaos of nosology" previously addressed in the history section of this paper in that there was so many different terms and uses of terms that uniformity simply did not exist. The 4th edition states that "major causalgia designates an extremely serious form of RSD produced by an injury to a major mixed nerve, usually in the proximal portion of the extremity", whereas, "minor causalgia designates a more common form of RSD produced by an injury to the distal part of the extremity involving a purely sensory branch of a nerve." The authors do acknowledge, however, that there are "other forms" of RSD that are "not associated with injury of a peripheral nerve".

Instructions for rating causalgia and RSD in the 4th edition follow uniformity. In other words, the two syndromes are not separated and have the same instructions. First, we are to rate any range of motion loss to any joints of the extremity. Then we are instructed to grade sensory deficits or pain and motor deficits (if the nerve has a motor function) and determine their respective severity multipliers. We are to then use the maximum percentage for the injured nerve in question and multiply the appropriate values representing the grades of severity of sensory and/or motor deficit previously determined.

Finally, we are instructed to combine the values of sensory rating, motor rating, and loss of range of motion to determine the final impairment rating.

The 4th edition approach is, therefore, valid for only causalgia from the historical perspective at least up until its book publication date in that the term is reserved for syndromes involving only an injury to a specific nerve. There is no role for impairment rating of RSD from the perspective of those who would define RSD at the time of publication as a pain syndrome that extended beyond the distribution of a single nerve.

The 5th edition was the first edition where the term "CRPS" actually appeared in the text. The 5th edition distinguished CRPS Type I from CRPS Type2 based upon whether the symptoms involved a specific nerve root or not. The 5th edition did a reasonable job of explaining recent research on the subject with regard to the fact that the sympathetic nervous system was not involved in the syndrome and that regional sympathetic nerve blockade had no role in the diagnosis. The authors went on to explain that their use of the term CRPS was based upon new insights into the constellation of symptoms, but went on to explain that an extensive differential diagnosis needed to be considered.

Great confusion regarding the methodology of determining impairment ratings was created because of internal inconsistency amongst the different chapters that addressed the topic.

The Upper Extremity Chapter explained that because the Guides is based upon objective findings primarily and that the differential diagnosis was considerable, a more conservative approach for impairment ratings was necessary than the diagnostic criteria that had been laid out by the IASP in 1994. Subsequently, the UE Chapter employed what is commonly referred to as the "Ensalada Table," named after Dr. Leon Ensalada who had offered a CRPS rating paradigm in a companion AMA text (The AMA Guides Casebook).[10] This table and paradigm mandated that at least 8 clinical or radiographic signs needed to be present concurrently at the time of the rating examination in order for the diagnosis of CRPS to be used for impairment rating purposes.

The instructions for CRPS ratings were quite different than in prior editions. Instead of limiting the rating process to identifiable nerve injury, the AMA Guides 5th introduced a protocol for rating CRPS Type I (comparing it to the prior term RSD), whereby the rating was simply a combination of any joint ROM loss with a purely subjective assignment of a percentage rating of the entire upper extremity from pain or sensory disturbance taken from table used to grade peripheral nerve disorders. For CRPS Type 2, the 5th edition continued the protocol of the 4th edition for causalgia, instructing the examiner to assign both grade values and percentage multipliers for both sensory and/or motor nerve involvement of a specific nerve and combining these values with any ROM loss.

The Neurology Chapter differed in its methodologies. The authors of the Neurology Chapter elected to continue to use the older terms RSD and causalgia and indicated that CRPS would specifically NOT be used because these "disorders" did not "represent a single diagnostic criterion." There is no instruction in the Neurology Chapter regarding a requirement for a certain amount of objective findings to be present, with a tendency for reliance in the text toward radiological findings and response to sympathetic block. It was as if the two chapter authors were living on a different planet.

To make matters even more confusing, the rating scheme in the Neurology Chapter rates upper extremity impairments higher for the dominant extremity, something that the UE Chapter does not.

The Lower Extremity Chapter discussion of CRPS does not help clear up any of the aforementioned inconsistencies. Rather, the LE Chapter discusses all terms (causalgia, reflex sympathetic dystrophy, and CRPS) but does not make a distinction between CRPS Type 1 and CRPS Type2. Amazingly, the LE Chapter states that "CRPS is further described in Section 13.8" when in fact, the authors of that Section specifically tell us why they are NOT describing CRPS. The methodology suggested for rating LE CRPS is to use the Lower Extremity Table that rates Station, Gait and Movement Disorders, and as is consistent with the Neurology Chapter, does not require a certain number of objective findings to be present. It should be noted that the rating process espoused by the Neurology Chapter (and defaulted into by the LE Chapter) has been criticized by the use of a wide range of numerical values for each impairment class. Some have therefore described this process as employing a strategy of "Exponential Subjectivity" when deriving a numerical impairment rating percentage.

Lastly, to add to the confusion, CRPS I appears as a ratable condition in the Pain Chapter of the 5th edition. The 5th edition pain chapter was the first to suggest that a numerical value impairment percentage could be assigned for pain alone. The authors of the Pain Chapter list CRPS Type I as a "well established pain syndrome without significant, identifiable organ dysfunction to explain the pain" and go on to state that it would therefore be a disorder that should be rated using the parameters within that chapter. The problem is that in order to use the Pain Chapter, other "rules" that are stated in the text include that these syndromes "are not ratable under the conventional rating system and also they do not fit any of the other chapters in the Guides." Contradictorily, there are 3 other chapters that do exactly that. Also, an inherent disconnect between rating percentages is created by inclusion of CRPS Type I in this Chapter in that the maximum whole person pain related rating allowed is 3%. In the experience of most, CRPS ratings using the other chapters are significantly higher than this.

Is there a way out of the 5th edition CRPS rating mess? Maybe. Dr. Ensalada was invited to author a clarification article which appeared in the AMA Guides Newsletter.[11] Unfortunately, the suggestion was akin to, "use what you feel is correct," amongst these different approaches. As could be expected, this bred continued disagreement and argumentative fodder especially within litigated claims.

The AMA Guides 6th edition brought with it a turn to a diagnostic approach toward impairment ratings. Much hope was expressed that the 6th edition would clarify some of the difficulties created by the 5th. It delivered on some, but not on others.

The 6th edition did eliminate the problem with internal inconsistency in that the UE and LE chapters agree on the methodology for rating CRPS Type I and CRPS Type II. Additionally, the diagnosis is not included in any of the other organ system chapters (Neurology and Pain specifically).

The 6th edition attempts to meld the updates to the CRPS diagnostic criteria commonly referred to as the "Budapest Criteria" that were published by a new IASP invitation only committee that tended towards a more liberal viewpoint,[12] with the older 5th edition "Ensalada Table" approach that turned an eye toward conservatism. Additional rules are included in the 6th edition for rating, such as: the requirement that the diagnosis has to be present for 1 year, that more than 1 physician must verify the diagnosis, that a comprehensive differential diagnostic process be undertaken.

In CRPS Type II, the AMA Guides 6th directs us to the peripheral nerve diagnosis based impairment tables which roughly correlate with other injuries or illnesses to the peripheral nervous system. Instructions tell the rating evaluator to determine the severity of the CRPS Type II based upon the approach for CRPS Type I which is to average the three adjustment factors for functional history, physical examination, and clinical studies. The severity must then be confirmed by the requisite number of objective criteria points obtained from a table listing such points (a reproduction of the "Ensalada Table" from the 5th ed.) and the class is adjusted if the objective points do not confirm the original calculated Class. Once the Class is determined, the severity of CRPS Type II is identified and found within the appropriate peripheral nerve DBI Table. An interesting dilemma that is not explained in the 6th edition is that non-key adjustment factors for the peripheral nerve ratings are then used only by application of the adjustments for functional history and clinical studies. This indicates that the physical examination defines the impairment values in the DBI table and, therefore, cannot be used as an adjustment factor; however, in the case of CRPS Type II, the physical examination non-key adjustment factor is used in the initial determination of the severity of Class of CRPS Type II.

The approach of the 6th edition for CRPS Type I is to base the severity of the class of impairment rating upon the average of the adjustment factors for functional history, physical examination, and clinical studies, with a "back up" confirmation based upon the number of objective diagnostic criteria points taken from the "Ensalada Table." Although this approach at first might seem more objective, critics have pointed out that a rating for CRPS under the 6th edition is actually easier to obtain as less objective criteria points are now needed compared to the UE Chapter 5th edition approach (4 versus 8 as a "cut-off" for use of the section)[13]. Additionally, they have pointed out that there is still inconsistency in that the initial verification of the CRPS diagnosis in the 6th edition is based upon the Budapest Criteria requiring only 2 objective signs whereas the impairment rating table states that the diagnosis is "not supportable" unless 4 such signs exist[13].

Where are we today? What we really need here is an honest admission that these various approaches have primary missed the mark. If we are to acknowledge and promote the concept that objective findings should rule over subjective reports, as the various AMA Guides texts would imply, there is an obvious problem with all editions approaches to CRPS Type I in particular with some spill over into CRPS Type II.

So what is a reasoned approach?

It seems reasonable to use a peripheral nerve based approach when we are evaluating a syndrome that likens itself to the current CRPS Type II in that the approach is no different than any other run of the mill peripheral nerve disorder evaluation. But, we would argue for abandonment of the term CRPS Type II in favor of simply referring to it as a peripheral nerve lesion with increased pain complaints.

In the case of the current syndrome referred to as CRPS Type I, we would advocate for use of a new term within impairment rating processes that has recently gained favor, "Amplified Musculoskeletal Pain Syndrome"[14-15]. Originally used in the pediatric literature to describe a variety of musculoskeletal pain syndromes[16], we suggest adoption of this term for the adult population undergoing impairment evaluations. Use of the term AMPS eliminates the majority of the confusion and difficulties that the concept of CRPS has created in the last two editions of the AMA Guides. By default, use of this term implies that there is indeed musculoskeletal pain that might be greater than expected, but avoids the scientific sideshow that is occurring regarding the CRPS controversy and returns the evaluation of all painful limbs to the origin of the Guides; in that, objectivity should rule the impairment rating process. By this strategy, any separate categorization or section within the Guides for a CRPS, or a like syndrome, is unnecessary. Use of the DBI (Diagnosis Based Impairment) methodology would be universal. Adjustments for non-key factors would be used to account for the additional burden of increased pain that these patients may have.

We recognize that adoption of this approach may have a consequence of lessening the claims of CRPS within the various compensation systems. Perhaps that is not an unworthy consideration given the significant controversy over the subject itself. Clinicians for a number of years have questioned the validity and voracity of CRPS claims and struggle immensely when considering the evidence based approach to a medical recommendation regarding its impact. There is nothing inherently wrong with redacting the diagnostic approach and subsequent impairment rating paradigm to a long accepted standard of extremity analysis, instead of continuing to promote a mystique-based view of ADL impact.

Section 8 References

1. Barth, RJ. A Historical Review of Complex Regional Pain Syndrome in the "Guides Library" and Broader Issues Raised by that History. The Guides Newsletter. November/December 2009. American Medical Association.

2. IASP. Classification of chronic pain: descriptions of chronic pain syndromes and definition of pain terms. 2nd ed. Seattle, WA: IASP Press; 1994.

3. Engelberg, AL. (editor) Guides to the Evaluation of Permanent Impairment, 3rd Edition Revised. 1990. American Medical Association.

4. Goede (editor) Guides to the Evaluation of Permanent Impairment, 4th Edition. 1993. American Medical Association.

5. Andersson GBJ, Cochiarella, L. (editors) Guides to the Evaluation of Permanent Impairment, 5th Edition. 2000. American Medical Association.

6. Rondinelli, RD et al. (editors) Guides to the Evaluation of Permanent Impairment, 6th Edition. 2008. American Medical Association.

7. Todorova J, Dantchev N, Petrova G. Complex regional pain syndrome acceptance and the alternative denominations in the medical literature. Med Princ Pract 2012;22:295–300.

8. Taylor, M. Past President AADEP, Chair of Texas Workers Compensation Commission Approved AADEP Training Courses (1992-2004) Personal Communication. 01-06-2014.

9. Lea, R. Past President AADEP, Lower Extremity Impairment Rating Instructor, Texas Workers Compensation Commission Approved AADEP Training Courses (1992-2002) Personal Communication. 05-15-2014.

10. Brigham CR (editor). The Guides Casebook. American Medical Association. 1999

11. Ensalada, LH. Fifth Edition: Causalgia, RSD, CRPS Impairment Evaluation. The Guides Newsletter. July/August 2001.

12. Harden RN, Bruehl S, Stanton-Hicks M, Wilson, PR. Proposed new diagnostic criteria for complex regional pain syndrome. Pain Med. 2007 May-Jun;8(4):326-31.

13. Martin DW. American Academy of Disability Evaluating Physicians. AMA Guides Sixth Edition Training Course (enduring material). Pain and Psychiatric Impairment Ratings. 2010

14. Cassidy, JT et al. (editors) Textbook of pediatric rheumatology (6th ed. ed.). Philadelphia: Saunders. 2011. p. 718

15. Rahimi H1, Siegel DM. A92: intensive physical therapy with desensitization in collaboration with psychological care is a successful outpatient treatment for amplified musculoskeletal pain syndrome. Arthritis Rheumatol. 2014 Mar;66 Suppl 11:S127

16. Sherry, DD. An overview of amplified musculoskeletal pain syndromes. J Rheumatol Suppl. 2000 Apr;58:44-8.

Section 9

Return to Function and Management of Dis/Ability

Complex Regional Pain Syndrome is a syndrome, meaning a collection of symptoms and findings seen together that lack clear medical explanation. Once the pathophysiology of a condition becomes known, it is typically renamed. Hence, "Down's Syndrome" became renamed as Trisomy 21. As a syndrome, CRPS probably is many different conditions that share some similar characteristics. Most cases involve the upper or the lower extremities. Most cases involve some degree of weakness, limited motion, and pain and/or numbness in a limb.

In the preceding section on treatment, physical therapy and/or occupational therapy have been recommended for decades both for prevention of CRPS after injury and for treatment of cases that occur. Exercise or use of the painful limb despite the pain felt during activity is generally part of the therapy program.

There is no published study indicating that exercise (therapy) has resulted in permanent worsening of objective findings in CRPS patients. Some studies have shown improvement with therapy (exercise)[1], while others have shown no benefit.[2]

Functional use of one's limbs is "exercise". Whether activities of daily living, or even work is being discussed, use of a limb is basically exercise of that limb.

If function is exercise, and if exercise is therapy/treatment for CRPS, then the syllogism is that function is treatment. Use of a limb with CRPS, whether for ADLs or for work, is treatment/therapy.

CRPS should be analyzed like any other condition for work ability assessment in terms of "risk", "capacity", and "tolerance".[3]

Risk is the basis on which physicians impose work restrictions, or prohibit the person from doing activities the individual actually can do, because of potential harm to self or others. In CRPS, there is no evidence of risk with work or activity in terms of objective worsening of the CRPS condition. In individuals with known partial injury to a peripheral nerve who do not develop CRPS Type II (for example, incomplete laceration of a nerve in the forearm), use of the limb does not pose risk. There is no "overuse of the remaining uninjured axons syndrome" postulated or reported. Exercise is prescribed hoping that use of the remaining functional axons will lead to hypertrophy and increased function in the still innervated motor units. Therefore, in CRPS type II, despite known nerve injury, exercise is therapy.

In CRPS Type I with no known nerve injury, there is no evidence that function despite pain makes the condition objectively worse.

Again, exercise (activity) is therapeutic. If the individual has limited use of a limb, the limited use may hinder activities. Thus, an individual who will not use the right lower limb because of a CRPS-like presentation should not be cleared to operate a vehicle where use of the right lower limb for foot controls is required (such as on a brake pedal). The disease or condition is not a basis for restrictions based on risk, but limited use may suggest activity restrictions based on risk assessment.

In CRPS, capacity may be an issue. For a police officer to be qualified to carry a weapon, the officer must be able to shoot satisfactorily with a pistol in each hand. With CRPS in an upper limb, the officer may not be able to produce a passing score on the pistol range qualifying exam. Officers must be able to maintain possession and control of a weapon during a physical struggle with a criminal. Individuals with CRPS Type I who won't use a limb fully, or who have nerve damage and CRPS Type II in a limb, should not be found fit to carry weapons. They would lack the capacity required.

Functional testing may show individuals with CRPS like presentations lack the current capacity to do heavier activity. However, symptom tolerance may be the basis for the limitations documented in functional testing, and not capacity. Whether an individual chooses to lift a 50 pound box during functional testing may be a reflection of symptom tolerance, and not of actual capacity to do the task.

Many individuals without CRPS who have been sedentary and who are hired into a physically demanding job lack the current measured capacity for all the job functions, and yet many successfully "toughen up" by using the job to build capacity over time. The greater the difference between the current capacity/tolerance on activity testing and the potential job demands in an individual with CRPS, the less likely the individual is to "toughen up" with a trial of return to work despite apparently lacking the required "capacity". Again, there is no published series of individuals with CRPS like presentations being made objectively worse by attempting activity or return to work, so permitting a trial of work or activity despite limited capacity is not a risk to the disease. A trial of return to work should be encouraged by those in whom risk appears not to be an issue, and whose functional testing appears adequate, or close to adequate, for job demands.

Tolerance is the ability of an individual to tolerate the symptoms of a condition during and after activity. Tolerance is a psychophysiological concept, and is not strictly biomedical. Many individuals work or participate in recreational sports despite pain from arthritis, prior injury, etc. Whether the benefits from the work or activity (pay, self-esteem, fun, etc.) are worth the "cost" of the symptoms, like pain and fatigue, is dependent on the value system of the individual and is not scientifically measureable. The decision on whether to use a limb with a CRPS-like presentation for work or recreational activity is an individual decision each CRPS patient ultimately must make. This is not a medical decision, and thus is not a question of risk assessment requiring a physician opinion, or comparison of capacity measurement to job descriptions for a physician opinion. **Tolerance decisions are a patient's decision**.

Patients with CRPS-like presentations may choose to work despite pain, or choose not to work, citing pain as their main reason. Physicians should remember that many people work every day despite pain, and that tolerance for pain issues is not a basis for a physician opinion that the individual should not work or is "disabled".

Chronic pain is frequent in adult populations and in people who work every day:

- In a population based study involving approximately 2000 working adults discovered that **only 13.2% of the participants reported being pain free at the beginning of the project.**[4]
- In a prospective study of over 4000 workers from industrial and service companies [Denmark] only 7.7% were free of pain at baseline and only 38% were **free** from **severe** pain.[5]

- The Gallop poll of U.S. adults in 2011 found that[6]
    - 31% have chronic neck or back pain
    - 26% have knee or leg pain, and
    - 18% have some other chronic pain.
    - **47% percent** of the adults had **at least one** of these chronic pain problems.

- The Institute of Medicine 2012 report "Relieving Pain in America" estimates **116,000,000** <u>adult</u> Americans have chronic pain.[7]

  - The 2012 U.S. <u>adult</u> population is estimated   at **228, 365,240**[8]
  - This would calculate at **just over 50% of adult Americans having chronic pain.**

Since pain cannot be objectively measured, and since chronic pain is very common, patients may say, "I don't want to work because of my pain." But, physicians should not certify disability because of pain when the work activity does not pose a "significant risk of substantial harm that is imminent"[9], and if the individual has the apparent capacity to do the required work tasks.

In summary, early after injury, once risk assessment concludes activity does not pose a risk to a limb still healing from injury, then gradual progressive exercise and work activity are generally prescribed as therapy for those with injury without CRPS- type presentations, and should also be prescribed for those with CRPS-type illness.

Section 9 References

1.   Oerlemans HM, Oostendorp RA, de Boo T, et al. Adjuvant physical therapy versus occupational therapy in patients with reflex sympathetic dystrophy/complex regional pain syndrome type I. Arch Phys Med Rehabil 2000; 81:49

2.   Oerlemans HM, Goris JA, de Boo T, Oostendorp RA. Do physical therapy and occupational therapy reduce the impairment percentage in reflex sympathetic dystrophy? Am J Phys Med Rehabil 1999; 78:533

3.   Talmage JB, Melhorn JM, Hyman MH. AMA Guides to the Evaluation of Work Ability and Return to Work. American Medical Association, Chicago, 2011.

4.   Kamaleri Y, Natvig B, Ihlebaek CM, Benth JS, Bruusgaard D. Change in the number of musculoskeletal pain sites: A 14-year prospective study. Pain. 2009 Jan;141(1-2):25-30]

5.   Andersen JH, Haahr JP, Frost P. A Two-Year Prospective Study of a General Working Population. *Arthritis & Rheumatism* 2007; 56 (4): 1355-1364

6.   http://www.gallup.com/poll/154169/chronic-pain-rates-shoot-until-americans-reach-late-50s.aspx   accessed 06/01/14

7.   Institute of Medicine. Relieving Pain in America: A Blueprint for Transforming Prevention, Care, Education, and Research. http://www.nap.edu/catalog.php?record_id=13172 or paperback ISBN 978-0-309-25627-8

8.   http://en.wikipedia.org/wiki/Demographics_of_the_United_States accessed 06/01/2014

9.   Americans with Disabilities Act legal standard- http://www.ada.gov/2010_regs.htm accessed 06/01/14

Section 10

Conclusion

This treatise is based largely on published, formalized conceptualizations of CRPS. The authors have the impression that there is a great discrepancy between such published conceptualizations and clinical practice, in that most such diagnoses in individual cases are not actually based on the utilization of any published conceptualization or diagnostic method. One author has collected hundreds of cases in which a diagnosis of CRPS was made. That process has produced the following observations: only two of the cases name the diagnostic method that was used in order to create the diagnosis; one of those two cases named a diagnostic method that does not actually exist ("the new AAPM criteria for CRPS"); the other one named one version of the Budapest protocol but did not actually document full utilization of even that flawed method; all other cases failed to mention any published diagnostic method (and yet a diagnosis of CRPS was claimed in each of those cases).

Similarly, another author has previously published a report, within an American Medical Association project, that most such diagnostic claims are made in the absence of a thorough differential diagnostic process. Consequently, the authors have the impression that clinical practice almost never adheres to the published conceptualizations of CRPS. The published conceptualizations of CRPS are, consequently, simply discussions of what someone thinks this construct should mean, rather than representing what such a diagnosis actually means in any individual case.

The authors strongly encourage termination of the long history of anti-scientific publications being produced which focus on what someone thinks the construct should mean. That history is to be replaced with scientific efforts focused on determining what a diagnosis of CRPS in any specific case actually means.

We believe strongly that the term CRPS should be abandoned by health care providers from their differential considerations regarding presentations of patients with painful extremities.

We hope to put to bed the debate on what "this is not" (it is not CRPS) and turn the focus instead towards "what this is."

APPENDIX A

Supplementary Information Regarding
Modern Diagnostic Protocols for Complex Regional Pain Syndrome

A. A continuing history of diagnostic chaos

Consistent with the ambiguous nature of the complex regional pain syndrome construct, and consistent the lack of scientific validity for the construct, there is no objective basis on which a diagnostic claim of complex regional pain syndrome can be based.[2-8,11-13,35]

Consequently, a variety of diagnostic protocols have been proposed which are based exclusively on description (rather than explanation, etiology, physiology, or any other aspects that are typical for general medical concepts which have been scientifically validated). Historically, such protocols have been "non-standardized, idiosyncratic, or incompatible"[23], and the existence of this multitude of protocols has highlighted the extreme unreliability of the complex regional pain syndrome construct.[4,13]

B. The International Association for the Study of Pain's original attempt to introduce some standardization

In 1994, the International Association for the Study of Pain (IASP) attempted to introduce some standardization through formal endorsement of a specific diagnostic protocol.[30]

However, that attempt was a failure on multiple levels. The 1994 IASP protocol has been subjected to much criticism, including criticism that was published directly by the IASP.[42] Aspects of the protocol which are vulnerable to criticism include its inherently self-defeating nature: it calls for complex regional pain syndrome to be excluded from diagnostic consideration if the case involves other potential explanations, such as a somatoform disorder or malingering, but it completely overlaps with diagnostic protocols for somatoform disorders, and most cases will overlap with the diagnostic protocol for malingering.[2] Clinicians and researchers continued to use competing diagnostic systems.[34,39] The protocol's adoption by scientists has been characterized as "sporadic at best".[1,25] Additional diagnostic protocols continued to emerge.[1,17,24,32,36,] Most importantly, field testing of the 1994 IASP protocol demonstrated that it leads to excessive diagnosis (diagnoses of complex regional pain syndrome being primarily applied to individuals who were known to not have complex regional pain syndrome).[20,24,25] This over-diagnosis problem was demonstrated to be so severe that a diagnosis of complex regional pain syndrome was found to be incorrect in the majority of research cases.[24]

As is discussed below, that 1994 IASP protocol was replaced in 2012.

C. The American Medical Association's first few attempts to overcome the shortcomings of the original IASP protocol

In spite of the lack of scientific validity for the concept of complex regional pain syndrome, the scientific and professional failure of the IASP's 1994 protocol, and the definitional lack of injury-relatedness for complex regional pain syndrome, the paradox of complex regional pain syndrome cases being dominated by legal claims (especially workers compensation claims) necessitated that the American Medical Association address this concept in its *Guides* Library.

The *Guides* Library's contributions to the discussion of the concept of complex regional pain syndrome apparently began with a 1997 *Guides Newsletter* article.[19] Because of the flawed nature of the 1994 IASP protocol (e.g. it's vulnerability to creating false diagnoses of complex regional pain syndrome), the 1997 article called for clinicians to avoid utilization of the IASP's protocol, in favor of an extensive differential diagnostic process seeking to eliminate alternative diagnoses (the specified differential diagnostic issues were all of a psychological nature: somatoform disorders, malingering, and factitious disorder), followed by objective determination of whether a list of physical signs and imaging findings were relevant to the examinee. In other words, a diagnostic approach was recommended which involved determining whether a recognizable syndrome of _objective_ findings emerged, in the context of a total lack of relevant alternative explanations for the clinical presentation. This was the beginning of a history of the *Guides* Library presenting protocols which attempted to remedy the inadequacy of the IASP's 1994 protocol (with the remainder of that history to be discussed later in this appendix). This protocol from the 1997 AMA article was re-emphasized in the AMA's 1999 *Guides Casebook*.[14]

An important element of the protocol that was recommended in the 1997 AMA article and the 1999 *Casebook* was the avoidance of any insinuation of injury-relatedness for complex regional pain syndrome-like presentations.

This avoidance of such insinuations contrasts against the impression of injury-relatedness that could be construed from the strange formatting of the 1994 IASP protocol.[30] The 1994 IASP protocol starts with the criterion, *"The presence of an initiating noxious event, or a cause of immobilization"*, but then strangely reverses itself by noting that this criterion is not actually required in order for a diagnosis of complex regional pain syndrome to be made. In contrast to that confusing set of circumstances and the insinuation of injury-relatedness that could be construed from it, the protocol that was recommended in the 1997 *Guides Newsletter* article did not contain any such language regarding an inciting event. This elimination of any misleading implication of injury-relatedness for the concept of complex regional pain syndrome was a precursor for research publications which indicated the need to abandon such implications[22], the development of other protocols which similarly removed insinuations of injury-relatedness[1,22,24,25,32,36] and for later *Guides* Library publications which highlighted the lack of injury-relatedness that is inherent to the concept of complex regional pain syndrome.[2,29,36]

The AMA approach was re-emphasized and expanded in the 2001 *Guides to the Evaluation of Permanent Impairment, 5*[th] *Edition.*[17] The *Guides 5*[th] *Edition* re-emphasized the directive for clinicians to avoid utilization of the IASP's protocol, in favor of an extensive differential diagnostic process seeking to eliminate alternative diagnoses (again specifying primary differential diagnostic issues which were all of a psychological nature), followed by objective determination of whether a list of physical signs and imaging findings applied to the examinee in the absence of relevant alternative diagnoses. The specifics of the protocol which had been presented in the previous *Guides* Library publications were expanded. The new protocol required a more conservative approach, by specifying that a longer list of objective findings needed to be present before a diagnosis of complex regional pain syndrome could be endorsed. That newly expanded protocol was the second major step in what would become a continuing process of the *Guides* Library presenting protocols which attempt to remedy the inadequacy of the IASP's 1994 protocol for complex regional pain syndrome, specifically including attempts to reduce the empirically established excessive diagnosis.

As is discussed below, that 2001 AMA protocol has been replaced.

D. Modern protocols

The above discussion of the history of IASP and AMA protocols did not include the details of those protocols, because they are all now obsolete. The following discussion provides a detailed discussion of the modern protocols which have replaced them (the following discussion is limited to the modern protocols which are most prominent in the United States).

There is a common element in all of the modern protocols: some adoption of criteria from what has been called "the Budapest protocol".

D. 1. The emergence of the Budapest protocol

"Budapest" refers to the city, in the Czech Republic, in which "a closed workshop (by invitation only) was held" in the fall of 2003, to discuss diagnostic and treatment considerations for complex regional pain syndrome.[24,25] The results of that closed meeting included an endorsement of a new protocol from the by-invitation- only group, and a proposal that the IASP consider adopting this new protocol (as is noted below, the IASP failed to adopt anything from this new protocol until 2012, and then only adopted portions of it).

The IASP published a book which was based on that "closed workshop".[42] That book reveals sponsorship of the "closed workshop" by a medical device manufacturer who stands to benefit financially from people receiving a diagnosis of complex regional pain syndrome. Personal communication with the reported primary organizer of the meeting confirmed such industry sponsorship of the meeting (Stanton- Hicks M. Personal communication, 12-2-2009). This is a concern, given aspects of the Budapest protocol which stray from the original IASP and AMA protocols in a manner that creates a risk of a severe exacerbation of the empirically established over-diagnosis of complex regional pain syndrome. Remarkably, the sponsorship by a commercial entity that will financially benefit from such over-diagnosis has not been acknowledged in more recent published discussions of the Budapest protocol.[25-27,31]

The Budapest protocol is largely based on research[15,22,24,26] that has been conducted in an effort to overcome the complete lack of scientific support for, and field test failures of, the 1994 IASP protocol. Although it contributes the significant benefit of avoiding the self-contradictory implication of injury-relatedness that was written into the 1994 IASP protocol, and adds a minimal level of quasi-scientific support, it is none-the-less afflicted by several significant concerns. Such concerns have repeatedly been published in AMA Guides Library and American Academy of Orthopaedic Surgeons publications[3,7,8] and are therefore only being discussed here in a highly summarized fashion. They include:

- The relevant research papers have been self-contradictory, misleading, and inaccurate in their use of the concepts of "sensitivity" and "specificity" for a health concept that the researchers acknowledge has no definitive diagnostic mechanism.[24,26] Therefore, the research reports of sensitivity, specificity, and diagnostic accuracy are consequently meaningless (see Section 3).

- The research designs that have been used for purposes of claiming some validation for the Budapest protocol are of a nature that can artificially inflate the resulting claims of diagnostic accuracy. This was acknowledged in an early research publication[24], but, as is the case for the early admission of corporate sponsorship, such acknowledgement of this flaw in the research design has been remarkably missing from more recent published discussions.[25-27,31]

- Despite this risk of producing artificially inflated claims of diagnostic accuracy, the results revealed that this protocol does not reliably distinguish between claims of complex regional pain syndrome, and cases that were specified as not involving complex regional pain syndrome.[24-26] The numbers are improved compared to similar research for the 1994 IASP protocol, but the research based on the Budapest protocol demonstrated that the diagnostic process is still unreliable, and the Budapest protocol continues the history of over-diagnosis. Furthermore, originally reported rates of diagnostic accuracy have decreased in later research.[26]

- The original research publications that reported some field testing of the Budapest protocol concluded with statements which specified that further attempts to validate the protocol were needed (in other words, the research design was not of a nature which credibly allowed for a claim that such research had produced validation for the protocol).[24,25] The more recent research-based claims of validation for the Budapest protocol involved the same almost meaningless research design that had been reported for prior research, and involved an emphasis on comparing the Budapest protocol to the 1994 IASP protocol.[26] None of this provides a sound basis for a claim of validation, given the inadequacies of the research design, and because the 1994 protocol was already known to be deeply flawed, unreliable, and a field test failure (and, consequently, could not serve as a credible contrast for attempting to validate the Budapest protocol). The resulting impression is that the original acknowledgement of a need for validation has been forgotten due to new research which is not actually capable of providing such validation.

- The research which has focused on the Budapest protocol has not been of a nature, in terms of design or results, that could actually validate the existence of a health condition that corresponds to the concept of complex regional pain syndrome.[13]

- The overlap with somatoform disorders and malingering that is inherent to the 1994 IASP protocol is repeated in the Budapest protocol (e.g. disproportionality, lack of diagnostic pathophysiology).

- The protocol involves an acknowledged reliance on the subjective reports of the examinee.[28]

- The protocol involves a misclassification of subjective examinee responses as objective signs (e.g. all of the following subjective issues which are dependent upon subjective reports or demonstrations from the examinee are mischaracterized within the protocols as "signs": hyperalgesia, allodynia, range of motion, weakness).[38]

- The protocol allows for examiner subjectivity to compromise the potential objective value of signs. For example, there is no requirement for abnormalities of temperature, skin color, sweating, or edema to be objectively evaluated. The protocol allows for all such issues to be subjectively evaluated by clinicians. Scientific findings have revealed that such subjective clinical impressions are not reliable, and are frequently inaccurate.[18,23,33,40]

- The Budapest protocol characterizes motor abnormalities as a diagnostic criterion for complex regional pain syndrome, in spite of scientific findings which have indicated that this issue is uniquely psychological when it occurs within the context of a complex regional pain syndrome claim.[41]

- The Budapest protocol was actually intentionally created to be two protocols – one for clinical work and a different one for scientific research.[24,25] If this aspect of the protocol is widely adopted, then the future of research on this subject will be largely irrelevant for health care. Because the clinical protocol is different from the research protocol, attempts to apply research findings to health care will be analogous to expecting that findings regarding apples will universally apply to oranges.

- The differential diagnostic requirement is softened (compared to the 1994 IASP and historical AMA protocols) in a manner that creates an even greater risk of excessive diagnosis than that which had been empirically demonstrated for the 1994 IASP protocol. Amazingly, the protocol also introduces an option of making a complex regional pain syndrome diagnosis in the absence of any diagnostic requirements, as is explained below.

- Published descriptions of the protocol do not agree with one another regarding the details of the protocol, even though the different versions of the protocol are both claimed as having been "adopted and codified" at the by-invitation-only, corporately sponsored meeting for purposes of "being proposed to the Committee for Classification of Chronic Pain of the IASP for inclusion in future revisions of their formal taxonomy and diagnostic criteria for pain states".[24,25] The authors have not found an explanation for this published contradiction regarding the details of the protocol.

Readers are strongly urged to keep the above limitations in mind as they review the following details of the Budapest protocol.[24,25] Because publications regarding the Budapest protocol are contradictory of one another in regard to the specifics of the protocol[24,25], the more recently published description is provided below, along with notes regarding contradictory information from the previously published description. Oddities of formatting (e.g. bold print, missing punctuation, etc.) are original to the source material.[25]

"Proposed clinical diagnostic criteria for CRPS

General definition of the syndrome:
CRPS describes an array of painful conditions that are characterized by a continuing (spontaneous and/or evoked) regional pain that is seemingly disproportionate in time or degree to the usual course of any known trauma or other lesion. The pain is regional (not in a specific nerve territory or dermatome) and usually has a distal predominance of abnormal sensory, motor, sudomotor, vasomotor, and/or trophic findings. The syndrome shows variable progression over time

To make the clinical diagnosis, the following criteria must be met:

1. Continuing pain, which is disproportionate to any inciting event

2. Must report at least one symptom in three of the four following categories:

> **Sensory:** *Reports of hyperesthesia and/or allodynia*

> **Vasomotor:** *Reports of temperature asymmetry and/or skin color changes and/or skin color asymmetry*

> **Sudomotor / Edema:** *Reports of edema and/or sweating changes and/or sweating asymmetry*

> **Motor / Trophic:** *Reports of decreased range of motion and/or motor dysfunction (weakness, tremor, dystonia) and/or trophic changes (hair, nail, skin)*

3. Must display at least one sign at time of evaluation in two or more of the following categories:

Sensory: Evidence of hyperalgesia (to pinprick) and/or allodynia (to light touch and/or temperature sensation and/or deep somatic pressure and/or joint movement)"

> (NOTE: The option for this sensory criterion to be satisfied by temperature sensation was missing from the 2005 publication, and then introduced without explanation in the 2007 publication, with both publications claiming that its version of this criterion had been "adopted and codified" at the closed meeting in Budapest in 2003.)

"Vasomotor: Evidence of temperature asymmetry (>1° C) and/or skin color changes and/or asymmetry"

> (NOTE: The requirement that temperature asymmetry must exceed one degree centigrade was missing from the 2005 publication, and then introduced without explanation in the 2007 publication, with both publications claiming that its version of this criterion had been "adopted and codified" at the closed meeting in Budapest in 2003.)

"Sudomotor / Edema: Evidence of edema and/or sweating changes and/or sweating asymmetry

Motor / Trophic: Evidence of decreased range of motion and/or motor dysfunction (weakness, tremor, dystonia) and/or trophic changes (hair, nail, skin)

4. There is no other diagnosis that better explains the signs and symptoms

For research purposes, diagnostic decision rule should be at least one symptom in all four symptom categories and at least one sign (observed at evaluation) in two or more sign categories."

The associated literature[25] specifies:

- *"Current distinctions between CRPS type I and CRPS type II subtypes, reflecting, respectively, the absence and presence of evidence of peripheral nerve injury, were retained".*

- *"A third diagnostic subtype called CRPS-NOS was recommended that would capture those patients who did not fully meet the new clinical criteria, but whose signs and symptoms could not better be explained by another diagnosis".*

Readers can note that the following two passages contribute to the increased risk of over- diagnosis that is associated with the Budapest protocol[25]:

- *"4. There is no other diagnosis that better explains the signs and symptoms."*

  This new wording can be compared to a corresponding passage from the1994 IASP protocol[30]: "This diagnosis is excluded by the existence of conditions that would otherwise account for the degree of pain and dysfunction." The new wording in the Budapest protocol puts the possibility of a diagnosis of complex regional pain syndrome on the same footing as any of the differential diagnostic issues, while the 1994IASP protocol emphasized the differential diagnostic issues had a preferential standing compared to the possibility of a complex regional pain syndrome diagnosis. This might not be a significant difference for any case in which a comprehensive differential diagnostic process is completed, because the overwhelmingly more common nature of many relevant differentials[5,6] will almost always result in the identification of another "diagnosis that better explains the signs and symptoms".

- *"A third diagnostic subtype called CRPS-NOS was recommended that would capture those patients who did not fully meet the new clinical criteria, but whose signs and symptoms could not better be explained by another diagnosis".*

- The risk of over-diagnosis is obvious in the above passage, as it indicates that a clinical presentation does not actually have to satisfy any diagnostic requirements in order for a complex regional pain syndrome diagnosis to be adopted. In competent clinical practice (involving a comprehensive differential diagnostic process), this might not be a significant issue, because the overwhelmingly more common nature of many relevant differentials[5,6] will almost always result in a realization that "signs and symptoms" can be better explained by "another diagnosis".

It is important to note that an early passage within this protocol (quoted above) specifies that the construct of complex regional pain syndrome is not intended to imply that a specific health condition has been identified, but is instead an umbrella construct which is potentially applicable to "an array of painful conditions". This is consistent with the historical purpose for which the complex regional pain syndrome construct was created. However, it is contradictory of other literature from authors of the published descriptions of the protocol, in that such other literature actually claims (without explanation) that the complex regional pain syndrome construct represents a single health condition.[27] This contradiction is another example of the pervasive unreliability of the complex regional pain syndrome construct.

D. 2. 2008: Criteria from the Budapest protocol are adopted for *the 6th Edition* of the AMA's *Guides to the Evaluation of Permanent Impairment*

2008 is the original copyright year for the 6th Edition of the *Guides to the Evaluation of Permanent Impairment*.[36] The *Guides 6th* continued the tradition of the AMA's *Guides* Library attempting to overcome the shortcomings of the 1994 IASP protocol for complex regional pain syndrome. In this regard, one of the versions of the criteria set from the clinical portion of the Budapest protocol was adopted, for the 6th Edition. This adoption was done in a fashion that was consistent with the *Guides* Library's historical emphasis on differential diagnosis (in other words, the Budapest protocol was not adopted in its published form from either 2005 or 2007).

This adoption of criteria set from the Budapest protocol by the *Guides 6th* appears to be the first endorsement, of any kind, of any aspect of the Budapest protocol by any health science academy. It also appears to be the first adoption of any aspect of the Budapest protocol by any entity that was not a recipient of the corporate sponsorship that led to the protocol's creation. Consistent with this impression, personal communication with the reported primary organizer of the Budapest "closed workshop" reported that he was not aware of any other endorsement of the protocol by any health science academy prior to this adoption of a criteria set for the *Guides 6th* (Stanton-Hicks M. Personal communication, 12-2-2009).

The 6th *Edition* incorporated criteria from one version of the Budapest clinical protocol for several reasons, including all of the following*:

- While the *Guides* 6th reiterates that complex regional pain syndrome has not been scientifically validated as an actual health condition, and the construct was created in a fashion which causes it to be inherently non-injury-related (and therefore, non-work-related), workers compensation claims and personal injury claims continue to dominate cases in which this diagnosis is utilized (and the purpose of the *Guides* is to assist administrators with such claims). The manner in which legal claims dominate diagnoses of complex regional pain syndrome indicated a need for the *Guides* 6th to address complex regional pain syndrome, in order to adhere to the impairment Guides goal of assisting claim administrators (e.g., judges, workers compensation commissions, etc.). Due to the paradox of this non-injury-related construct being dominated by occupational injury legal claims, the only means by which the contributors to the 6th *Edition* (including the author of this appendix) could construe a workers compensation-relevant example was to discuss a scenario in which an assumption of work-relatedness was mistakenly forced onto the case by administrative officials (since there would not be any credible basis for concluding work-relatedness).

*The author is reporting the following based on his direct experience as a contributor and reviewer for the *Guides 6th*, including contributing to the creation of the *Guides 6th* discussions of complex regional pain syndrome

- Although the scientific "validation" research that has been conducted for the Budapest protocol is largely misleading and meaningless (as was discussed above, and is more fully discussed in the Borchers review, and in other sections of this paper), its existence provides a basis for claiming that the Budapest criteria has been subjected to more study than prior criteria sets.

- The Budapest criteria avoids the self-contradictory insinuations of injury- relatedness that had compromised the 1994 IASP criteria.

- Reviewers/contributors who were involved in the creation of the *Guides 6th* predicted that the Budapest criteria would eventually be more widely utilized within health care than other criteria sets would be, and, consequently, the *Guides 6th* would have the best chance of being consistent with health care long-term if it utilized the Budapest criteria in some manner (even if the *Guides 6th* did so in a fashion that avoided the risk of increased excessive diagnosis that was inherent in the originally published versions of the Budapest protocol).

In order to avoid non-scientific claims, the *Guides 6th* did not adopt the "General definition" portion of the Budapest protocol. Instead, the *Guides 6th* provided a far more extensive discussion which emphasizes all of the following...

- the lack of scientific credibility for the complex regional pain syndrome construct
- the construct's inherent lack of injury-relatedness

- the role of disuse in the creation of relevant presentations

- the unreliable nature of a diagnostic claim of complex regional pain syndrome
- the necessity of a comprehensive differential diagnostic process

- the greater importance of differential diagnosis relative to diagnostic criteria

- the necessary elimination of complex regional pain syndrome from diagnostic consideration if any potentially relevant differential cannot be ruled out

- almost all differential diagnostic issues are far more probable than complex regional pain syndrome is said to be

The *Guides* 6th introduced several mechanisms for the purpose of minimizing the increased risk of excessive diagnosis that is inherent to the Budapest protocol:

- The *Guides* 6th did not accept the complex regional pain syndrome NOS concept (as was discussed above, this is the "subtype", from the Budapest protocol, which allowed a complex regional pain syndrome diagnosis to be made for cases which did not satisfy diagnostic requirements for type one or type two).

- Because of the lack of scientific credibility for the concept of complex regional pain syndrome, and because almost all differential diagnosis issues are going to be far more common than complex regional pain syndrome is said to be[5,6], and because all of the objective physical findings that have been written into the concept of complex regional pain syndrome can be created simply through disuse of the involved body part[16], the 6th Edition specifies that the criteria set from the Budapest protocol is only to be utilized after a comprehensive differential diagnostic process has been completed in a fashion that rules out all differentials. By emphasizing the necessity of such a differential diagnostic process, the 6th Edition largely overcomes the increased vulnerability to excessive diagnosis of complex regional pain syndrome that is otherwise built into the Budapest protocol.

In regard to that differential diagnostic requirement, the *Guides* 6th references another American Medical Association publication[5] which emphasizes that, at a minimum, the list of differential diagnostic issues which must be evaluated for and ruled out before a complex regional pain syndrome diagnosis can be credible, includes (but is not limited to):

- psychopathology that would have traditionally fallen into the category of somatoform disorders
- factitious disorder
- malingering
- personality disorders
- psychopathology that would have traditionally fallen into the category of anxiety disorders
- psychopathology that would have traditionally fallen into the category of mood disorders
- psychopathology that would have traditionally fallen into the category of substance-related disorders
- psychotic disorders
- Raynaud's phenomenon/disease
- cellulitis
- thromboangiitis obliterans
- thrombosis
- traumatic vasospasm
- nerve entrapment
- herpes zoster
- rheumatologic conditions
- stress fracture
- diabetic neuropathy

If a comprehensive differential diagnostic process rules out all potential differentials, then the *Guides 6th* calls for a version of the Budapest criteria to be applied to the clinical presentation. The criteria set which is presented in the *Guides 6th* is as follows:

1. Continuing pain, which is disproportionate to any inciting event

2. Must report at least 1 symptom in 3 of the 4 following categories:

Sensory: Reports of hyperesthesia and/or allodynia

Vasomotor: Reports of temperature asymmetry and/or skin color changes and/or skin color asymmetry

Sudomotor / Edema: Reports of edema and/or sweating changes and/or sweating asymmetry

Motor / Trophic: Reports of decreased range of motion and/or motor dysfunction (weakness, tremor, dystonia) and/or trophic changes (hair, nail, skin)

3. Must display at least 1 sign at time of evaluation in 2 or more of the following categories:

Sensory: Evidence of hyperalgesia (to pinprick) and/or allodynia (to light touch and/or deep somatic pressure and/or joint movement)

Vasomotor: Evidence of temperature asymmetry and/or skin color changes and/or asymmetry

Sudomotor / Edema: Evidence of edema and/or sweating changes and/or sweating asymmetry

Motor / Trophic: Evidence of decreased range of motion and/or motor dysfunction (weakness, tremor, dystonia) and/or trophic changes (hair, nail, skin)

4. There is no other diagnosis that better explains the signs and symptoms

This criteria set follows the 2005 published version of the Budapest protocol more closely than the 2007 version in the following ways:

- Temperature sensation has not been included as a physical examination tool that can be used for the hyperalgesia criterion.

- The requirement that a finding of temperature asymmetry must exceed 1°C in order to satisfy the relevant diagnostic requirement was not included.

D. 3. 2008: A modified utilization of the Budapest criteria set is adopted for the American College of Occupational and Environmental Medicine's *Occupational Medicine Practice Guidelines*

2008 is also listed as the year in which a revision was undertaken for the American College of Occupational and Environmental Medicine's (ACOEM) *Occupational Medicine Practice Guidelines* chapter which is entitled "Chronic Pain".[1]

A pre-publication draft of that chapter was circulated for review, and the American Academy of Neurology asked one of the authors of this paper to represent it in that review process. That pre-publication draft included endorsement of the criteria set from the Budapest protocol in a form that included an increased risk of excessive diagnosis. The written response to reviewing that chapter provided to the American Academy of Neurology advised of the need to highlight the corporate sponsorship and associated financial conflict of interest that was associated with the Budapest protocol, and the consequent increased risk of excessive diagnosis that was inherent to that protocol.

The American Academy of Neurology shared that recommendation with ACOEM, and the editor-in-chief of the ACOEM *Guidelines* consequently solicited assistance in developing a manner in which those *Guidelines* could help to minimize the risk of excessive diagnosis. Efforts in this regard led to a modification of the differential diagnosis language from the protocol (see item #4 below), so that it was more consistent with the 1994 IASP protocol and with the 6*th* Edition of the AMA's *Guides to the Evaluation of Permanent Impairment*.

The ACOEM protocol also rejected the complex regional pain syndrome NOS subtype from the Budapest protocol.

The ACOEM protocol also differs from the Budapest protocol in that the "General Definition" portion of the Budapest protocol was not adopted.

The ACOEM protocol is consistent with the 2005 criteria set that was published for the Budapest protocol, and the 6th Edition of the AMA's impairment Guides. The ACOEM criteria set does not match the 2007 version of the Budapest protocol, in that the following issues were not included: temperature sensation as a physical examination tool that can be used for the hyperalgesia criterion; the requirement that a finding of temperature asymmetry must exceed 1°C in order to satisfy the relevant diagnostic requirement.

The resulting ACOEM criteria reads as follows:

1. Continuing pain, which is disproportionate to the inciting event

2. At least one symptom in three of these four categories:

Sensory: hyperesthesia and/or allodynia

Vasomotor: temperature asymmetry and/or skin color changes and/or skin color asymmetry

Sudomotor / edema: edema and/or sweating changes and/or sweating asymmetry

Motor / trophic: decreased range of motion and/or motor dysfunction
(weakness, tremor, dystonia) and/or trophic changes (hair, nail, skin)

3. At least one sign at time of evaluation in two or more of the following categories:

Sensory: evidence of hyperalgesia to pinprick and/or allodynia to light touch and/or deep somatic pressure and/or joint movement

Vasomotor: Evidence of temperature asymmetry and/or skin color changes and/or asymmetry

Sudomotor / edema: evidence of edema and/or sweating changes and/or sweating asymmetry

Motor / trophic: evidence of decreased range of motion and/or motor dysfunction (weakness, tremor, dystonia) and/or trophic changes (hair, nail, skin)

4. Diagnosis: CRPS is excluded by the existence of conditions that would otherwise account for the degree of pain and dysfunction.

The ACEOM *Guidelines* warn that the above criteria set "may be inadequate" because it fails to mention objective measurement of the supposed "signs". Consequently, within the ACOEM *Guidelines*, objective measurement of such signs is "required"; the *Guidelines* offer examples such as temperature probes and volumetry.

Consistent with the emphasis on psychological differentials from the 6th *Edition* of the AMA's impairment *Guides* and all prior relevant *Guides* Library publications, the ACOEM *Guidelines* also report: "The threshold for concomitant psychological consultation and psychometric testing in such circumstances should be quite low."

D. 4. 2012: A modified utilization of the Budapest criteria set is adopted by the International Association for the Study of Pain

While the 2003 "closed workshop" in Budapest was reportedly focused on recommending the Budapest protocol for adoption by the International Association for the Study of Pain (IASP)[24,25], the IASP has not adopted the protocol, and did not even adopt the criteria set from the Budapest protocol until 2012.[31]

The 2012 IASP protocol has the following characteristics:

- The "General Definition" portion of the original version of the Budapest protocol[25,26] has been eliminated in favor of a more expansive discussion.

- The use of temperature sensation as a physical examination tool for the hyperalgesia criterion, which is part of the 2007 published version of the Budapest protocol was not adopted, therefore making it consistent with the 2005 publication of the Budapest protocol, and with the AMA and ACEOM versions of that criterion.

- The requirement that a finding of temperature asymmetry must exceed 1°C in order to satisfy the relevant diagnostic requirement, which is part of the 2007 published version of the Budapest protocol was not adopted, again consistent with the 2005 publication of the Budapest protocol, and with the AMA and ACEOM versions of that criterion.

- The complex regional pain syndrome NOS subtype from the Budapest protocol is included in the IASP version, thereby allowing a complex regional pain syndrome diagnosis to be made in cases which do not satisfy any diagnostic requirements for type one or type two.

- The differential diagnosis criterion is of a nature that is consistent with the 2005 and 2007 publications of the Budapest protocol, and consequently eliminates the historical IASP and AMA principle that complex regional pain syndrome was excluded from diagnostic consideration by the presence of any other issues which could explain the clinical presentation. Like the inclusion of the complex regional pain syndrome NOS subtype, this element of the modern IASP protocol increases the risk of excessive diagnosis that was empirically established for the 1994 IASP protocol.

- The 2012 IASP protocol provides a differential diagnostic discussion which is remarkably minimal compared to the AMA and American Academy of Orthopaedic Surgeons discussions.[5,6,36] The IASP discussion in this regard fails to consider most of the strongest scientific findings, such as the prominence of legal claims among people who obtain a complex regional pain syndrome diagnosis[9,10,38], the prominence of personality disorders and other pre-existing forms of psychopathology among people who obtain a complex regional pain syndrome diagnosis[5,6,9,10] , and the prominence of people who obtain a complex regional pain syndrome diagnosis responding to objective assessment in a manner that indicates an invalid clinical presentation.[21] In fact, the IASP discussion inexplicably avoids consideration of most of the scientific findings that have been discussed in relevant AMA and American Academy of Orthopaedic Surgeons publications[5,6,9,10] As such, the minimal nature of the IASP 2012 differential diagnosis discussion appears to be a continuation of the anti-scientific approach which has been a feature of the construct from the time of its creation.

- The three bullet points directly above indicate that the 2012 IASP protocol creates an extreme risk of excessive diagnosis, including a greater risk than the risk that was created by the 1994 IASP protocol, which reportedly prompted the creation of the Budapest protocol because it was demonstrated to be so vulnerable to over-diagnosis that field trials revealed most complex regional pain syndrome diagnoses to be false.

- The 2012 IASP protocol strays from the Budapest protocol's distinction between complex regional pain syndromes type one and type two. The difference between the IASP and Budapest protocols in this regard is demonstrated by a comparison of these two passages:

  o 2007 published discussion of the Budapest protocol:

    - "Current distinctions between CRPS type I and CRPS type II subtypes, reflecting, respectively, the absence and presence of evidence of peripheral nerve injury, were retained".[25]

    This is notably different from the IASP emphasis, quoted below, on "a major nerve lesion" which does not need to be of a peripheral nature.

o 2012 IASP version:

- "CRPS I ...As defined above." (referring to the descriptive "DiagnosticCriteria" section quoted below, and all other portions of the 2012 IASP discussion except for the section labeled "Differential Diagnosis")

- "CRPS II ... Defined as above with electrodiagnostic or physical evidence of a major nerve lesion."

  This is notably different from the Budapest version, quoted above, which requires the nerve lesion to be of a peripheral nature, but which does not require any aspect of the lesion to be "major".

The 2012 IASP adoption of a modification of the criteria set from the Budapest protocol reads as follows:

"Diagnostic Criteria

There are two versions of the diagnostic criteria: A clinical version meant to maximize diagnostic sensitivity with adequate specificity, and a research version meant to more equally balance optimal sensitivity and specificity.

Clinical Diagnostic Criteria for CRPS

1) *Continuing pain, which is disproportionate to any inciting event.*

2) *Must report at least one symptom in three of the four following categories:*

Sensory: Reports of hyperalgesia and/or allodynia.

Vasomotor: Reports of temperature asymmetry and/or skin color changes and/or skin color asymmetry.

Sudomotor/Edema: Reports of edema and/or sweating changes and/or sweating asymmetry.

Motor/Trophic: Reports of decreased range of motion and/or motor dysfunction(weakness, tremor, dystonia) and/or trophic changes (hair, nails, skin).

3) *Must display at least one sign* at time of evaluation in two or more of the following categories:*

Sensory: Evidence of hyperalgesia (to pinprick) and/or allodynia (to light touch and/or deep somatic pressure and/or joint movement).

Vasomotor: Evidence of temperature asymmetry and/or skin color changes and/or asymmetry.

Sudomotor/Edema: Evidence of edema and/or sweating changes and/or sweating asymmetry.

Motor/Trophic: Evidence of decreased range of motion and/or motor dysfunction(weakness, tremor, dystonia) and/or trophic changes (hair, nails, skin).

4) *There is no other diagnosis that better explains the signs and symptoms.*

A sign is counted only if it is observed at time of diagnosis.

**Research criteria for CRPS are recommended that are more specific, but less sensitive than the clinical criteria; they require that four of the symptom categories and at least two sign categories be present.*

Subtypes of CRPS

CRPS I (old name: Reflex Sympathetic Dystrophy): As defined above.

CRPS II (old name: Causalgia): Defined as above with electrodiagnostic or physical evidence of a major nerve lesion.

CRPS-NOS (Not Otherwise Specified): Partially meets CRPS criteria, not better explained by any other condition."*

Readers can also note the following confusing elements of the 2012 IASP protocol. The passage which reads "CRPS I (old name: Reflex Sympathetic Dystrophy)" could be misconstrued as an indication that complex regional pain syndrome type one and reflex sympathetic dystrophy are new and old names for the same construct, when in fact, the construct of complex regional pain syndrome type one is drastically different from the discontinued construct of reflex sympathetic dystrophy. The passage which reads "CRPS II (old name: Causalgia)" could be misconstrued as an indication that the concept of causalgia has been discontinued in favor of complex regional pain syndrome type two, when in fact, the IASP's system[31] actually maintains causalgia as a diagnostic entity.

D. 5. 2013: *ODG Treatment in Workers Compensation* references the 2007 version of the Budapest criteria set.

In 2013, the guidelines within *ODG Treatment in Workers Comp* were modified to include referencing of the 2007 version of the Budapest criteria set. Key issues from the ODG text[32] include:

- An emphasis on differential diagnosis, consistent with the emphasis in this regard from the AMA[5,36], American Academy of Orthopaedic Surgeons[6], and American College of Occupational and Environmental Medicine literature.[1] This emphasis is markedly different (more thorough) than the versions of the Budapest protocol[24,25] and the modern IASP protocol.[31] Relevant passages from *ODG Treatment* include:

    o "Financial gain (such as that involved with litigation) has been found to increase the risk of CRPS."

    o "There should be evidence that all other diagnoses have been ruled out. A diagnosis of CRPS should not be accepted without a documented and complete differential diagnostic process completed as a part of the record."

    o "It is suggested that in the absence of a differential diagnostic evaluation for patients with a suggested diagnosis of CRPS, management can be abortive and iatrogenic harm may follow."

    o "The importance of establishing a correct diagnosis and to prevent potentially harmful and/ or unwarranted treatment cannot be emphasized enough."

    o "the objective physical signs of CRPS, including imaging, can be created with disuse and or physical manipulation."

- While the overall approach of the 2005 or 2007 versions of the Budapest protocol was not adopted into *ODG Treatment,* a criteria set reportedly based on the Budapest protocol was "recommended", and the text specifically recommends the 2007 version of that set, including the use of temperature sensation for the sensory "sign" criterion and the requirement that the temperature asymmetry sign involve a discrepancy of greater than one degree centigrade.

- In regard to the complex regional pain syndrome NOS diagnosis, the ODG text specifies: "This diagnosis is not endorsed by ODG."

The new ODG criteria set parallels the criteria from the 2007 version of the Budapest protocol, and specifically reads as follows:

"The diagnostic criteria are the following: (1) Continuing pain, which is disproportionate to any inciting event; (2) Must report at least one symptom in three of the four following categories: (a) Sensory: Reports of hyperesthesia and/or allodynia; (b) Vasomotor: Reports of temperature asymmetry and/or skin color changes and/or skin color asymmetry; (c) Sudomotor/Edema: Reports of edema and/or sweating changes and/or sweating asymmetry; (d) Motor/Trophic: Reports of decreased range of motion and/or motor dysfunction (weakness, tremor, dystonia) and/or trophic changes (hair, nail, skin); (3) Must display at least one sign at time of evaluation in two or more of the following categories: (a) Sensory: Evidence of hyperalgesia (to pinprick) and/or allodynia (to light touch and/or temperature sensation and/or deep somatic pressure and/or joint movement); (b) Vasomotor: Evidence of temperature asymmetry (>1°C) and/or skin color changes and/or asymmetry; (c) Sudomotor/Edema: Evidence of edema and/or sweating changes and/or sweating asymmetry; (d) Motor/Trophic: Evidence of decreased range of motion and/or motor dysfunction (weakness, tremor, dystonia) and/or trophic changes (hair, nail, skin); (4) There is no other diagnosis that better explains the signs and symptoms."

Appendix A References:

1. American College of Occupational and Environmental Medicine. Chronic Pain (Revised 2008), In: *Occupational Medicine Practice Guidelines, 2nd Edition.* American College of Occupational and Environmental Medicine, 2008.

2. Barth, RJ, and Bohr, TW. Challenges in the IASP's Diagnostic Conceptualization for CRPS-1 (Formerly Conceptualized as RSD), Part 1. *The Guides Newsletter.* January/February, 2006a. American Medical Association.

3. Barth, RJ, and Bohr, TW. Challenges in the IASP's Diagnostic Conceptualization for CRPS-1 (Formerly Conceptualized as RSD), Part 2. *The Guides Newsletter.* March/April, 2006b. American Medical Association.

4. Barth, RJ. Complex Regional Pain Syndrome (CRPS): Unratable through the PainChapter. *The Guides Newsletter.* July/August, 2006. American Medical Association.

5. Barth RJ and Haralson R. Differential Diagnosis for Complex Regional Pain Syndrome.*The Guides Newsletter,* September/October 2007a. American Medical Association.

6. Barth RJ and Haralson R. Differential Diagnosis for Complex Regional Pain Syndrome. In: Melhorn JM and Shields NN. *9th Annual Occupational Orthopaedics and Workers Compensation: A Multidisciplinary Perspective.* 2007b. American Academy ofOrthopaedic Surgeons.

7. Barth RJ. A Historical Review of CRPS in The American Medical Association's Guides Library. *The Guides Newsletter,* November/December, 2009. American Medical Association.

8. Barth RJ. A Historical Review of CRPS in The American Medical Association's Guides Library. In: Melhorn JM and Talmage JB. *13th Annual American Academy of Orthopaedic Surgeons Occupational Orthopaedics and Workers Compensation: A Multidisciplinary Perspective.* 2011. American Academy of Orthopaedic Surgeons.

9. Barth RJ. Chronic Pain: Fundamental Scientific Considerations, Specifically for Legal Claims. *AMA Guides Newsletter*, Jan/Feb 2013. American Medical Association.

10. Barth RJ. Chronic Pain: Fundamental Scientific Considerations, Specifically For Legal Claims. In: Melhorn JM (editor). *16th Annual AAOS Workers' Compensation and Musculoskeletal Injuries: Improving Outcomes with Back-to-Work, Legal and Administrative Strategies.* 2014. American Academy of Orthopaedic Surgeons.

11. Bass C. Complex regional pain syndrome medicalises limb pain. British Medical Journal. 2014 Apr 28;348:g2631.

12. Biller, J (Chair), et al. Neuropathic pain and Iatrogenesis. Pages 91-104 in: IatrogenicNeurology, Continuum, 7, 2, 2001. American Academy of Neurology.

13. Borchers AT, Gershwin ME. Complex regional pain syndrome: A comprehensive and critical review. Autoimmun Rev. 2013 Oct 23.

14. Brigham CR (editor). *The Guides Casebook.* American Medical Association, 1999.

15. Bruehl S, Harden RN, Galer BS, Saltz S, Bertram M, Backonja M, Gayles R, Rudin N,Bhugra MK, and Stanton-Hicks M. External validation of IASP diagnostic criteria forComplex Regional Pain Syndrome and proposed research diagnostic criteria. *Pain* 1999;81:147-154.

16. Butler SH: Disuse and CRPS, in Harden RN, Baron R, Janig W (eds): *Complex RegionalPain Syndrome*. Seattle, WA: IASP Press, 2001, pp 141-150.

17. Cocchiarella, L. and Anderson, G. (editors) (2001). *Guides to the Evaluation ofPermanent Impairment, Fifth Edition*. American Medical Association.

18. Dijkstra PU, van der Schans CP, Geertzen JH. Risk perception of developing complex regional pain syndrome-1. Clin Rehabil2003 ;17(4):944-6.

19. Ensalada LH. The Challenge of Evaluating RSD Impairment and Disability (Part 1).Guides Newsletter, November/December, 1997. Pages 3-5.

20. Galer BS, Bruehl S, Harden RN. IASP diagnostic criteria for Complex Regional PainSyndrome: a preliminary empirical validation study. Clin J Pain 1998; 14:48-54.

21. Greiffenstein M, Gervais R, Baker WJ, Artiola L, Smith H. Symptom validity testing in medically unexplained pain: a chronic regional pain syndrome type 1 case series. *Clin Neuropsychol*. 2013;27(1):138-47.

22. Harden RN, Bruehl S, Galer BS, et al. Complex regional pain syndrome: are the IASPdiagnostic criteria valid and sufficiently comprehensive? *Pain*, 83 (1999), 211-219.

23. Harden RN, Baron R, Janig W, editors. *Complex Regional Pain Syndrome*. Seattle: International Association for the Study of Pain Press; 2001.

24. Harden, RN, and Bruehl, SP. Diagnostic Criteria: The Statistical Derivation of the Four Criterion Factors. In: Wilson, PR, Stanton-Hicks, M, and Harden, RN. *CRPS: Current Diagnosis and Therapy*. International Association for the Study of Pain, Seattle: 2005.

25. Harden RN, Bruehl S, Stanton-Hicks M, Wilson PR. Proposed new diagnostic criteria for complex regional pain syndrome. *Pain Med.* 2007 May-Jun;8(4):326-31.

26. Harden RN, Bruehl S, Perez RSGM, et al. Validation of proposed diagnostic criteria (the"Budapest Criteria") for Complex Regional Pain Syndrome. *Pain*, 150 (2010a) 268–274.

27. Harden RN & Bruehl S. Complex Regional Pain Syndrome. Chapter 25 in: Fishman SM, Ballantyne JC, & Rathmell JP (editors). Bonica's Management of Pain, Fourth Edition. Lippincott Williams & Wilkins, 2010b.

28. Harden RN. Objectification of the diagnostic criteria for CRPS. Pain Med. 2010c Aug;11(8):1212-5.

29. Melhorn JM, Ackerman WE (editors). *Guides to the Evaluation of Disease and Injury Causation.* American Medical Association, 2008.

30. Merskey H, & Bogduk N (editors). *Classification of Chronic Pain, Second Edition.* International Association for the Study of Pain, 1994.

31. Merskey H, & Bogduk N (editors). *Classification f Chronic Pain, Second Edition(Revised).* International Association for the Study of Pain, 2012.

32. ODG Treatment in Workers Comp: http://www.odg-twc.com/ accessed 10/01/2014

33. Oerlemans HM, Perez RS, Oostendorp RA, et al. Objective and subjective assessments of temperature differences between the hands in reflex sympathetic dystrophy. *Clin Rehabil* 1999;13(5):43-8.

34. Reinders MF, Geertzen JH, Dijkstra PU. Complex regional pain syndrome type I: use of the International Association for the Study of Pain diagnostic criteria defined in 1994. *Clinical Journal of Pain.* 2002; 18: 207-15.

35. Ring D, Barth R, and Barsky A. Evidence-based medicine: disproportionate pain and disability, *Journal of Hand Surgery*, volume 34a, August 2010, 1345-1347.

36. Rondinelli RD, Brigham CR, Genovese E, et al. (Editors). *Guides to the Evaluation of Permanent Impairment Sixth Edition (Second Printing).* American Medical Association, 2009.

37. Sandroni P, Benrud-Larson LM, McClelland RL, and Low PA. Complex regional pain syndrome, type I: incidence in Olmsted County, a population-based study. Pain 2003; 103: 199-207.

38. Talmage JB, Melhorn JM, Ackerman WE, & Barth RJ. Musculoskeletal Disorders: Conditions of Uncertain Pathophysiology – Acute and Chronic Pain, in: Melhorn, JM, et al. (editors). *Guides to the Evaluation of Disease and Injury Causation, Second Edition.* 2013. American Medical Association.

39. van de Beek WJ, Schwartzman RJ, van Nes SI. Diagnostic criteria used in studies of reflex sympathetic dystrophy. *Neurology* 2002, 58 (4): 522-6.

40. van de Vusse AC, Stomp-van den Berg SG, de Vet HC, Weber WE. Interobserver reliability of diagnosis in patients with complex regional pain syndrome. Eur J Pain.2003;7(3):259-65.

41. Verdugo RJ, Ochoa JL. Abnormal movements in complex regional pain syndrome:assessment of their nature. *Muscle Nerve.* 2002; 23 (2): 198-205.

42. Wilson, PR, and Bogduk, N. Retrospection, Science and Epidemiology. In: Wilson, PR, Stanton-Hicks, M, and Harden, RN. *CRPS: Current Diagnosis and Therapy.* International Association for the Study of Pain, Seattle: 2005.

CPSIA information can be obtained at www.ICGtesting.com
Printed in the USA
LVOW06s1523231215

467565LV00002B/3/P